Heal Yourself and Your Loved Ones

Home Massage Therapy

Book 1

Heal Yourself and Your Loved Ones

Home Massage Therapy Book 1

Healing Society, Inc.
7664 W. Lake Mead Blvd. # 109
Las Vegas, NV 89128

e-mail: book@healingsociety.org
Web site: www.healingplaza.com

If you are unable to order this book from your local bookseller,
you may order directly from the publisher.
Call 1-877-324-6425, toll-free.

Library of Congress Control Number: 2004104232
ISBN: 0-9720282-9-3

Translated by Alexander Choi and Julie Han
at Dahn Healing Institute
Designed by Pishion
Printed in South Korea

Heal Yourself and Your Loved Ones

Home Massage Therapy

Book 1

DAHN HEALER SCHOOL

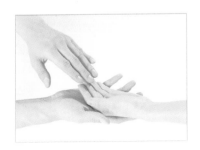

Healing Society

Preface

Many in this world are in search of magical medicines and renowned healers, but only few know the importance and benefits of the natural healing powers one has within oneself. Health is very closely within our reach. Dahnhak does not seek remedies from afar. It researches and develops programs to aid all individuals to easily discover natural self-healing mechanisms from within. Dahnhak Meridian Exercise, Dahn-Jon Breathing, Dahn-Diet, and meditation are all methods of improving circulation of 'Ki-energy' in our bodies, and to enhance our self-healing power.

Dahnhak Hwal-Gong is a healing method that does not require special training or skills. Anybody can utilize these life-supporting principles on a daily basis. By simply laying your bare hands on someone to heal you can open the hearts and minds of your family, neighbors and friends, and come to know the pure joy in giving and receiving love. Perhaps, today, we rely too much on synthesized medicine. We deprive ourselves of knowing the power of touch that transmits our loving warmth and devotion.

If you are suffering from being misunderstood by your friends and family, we recommend that you try Dahnhak Hwal-Gong. When your body is in pain there is nothing that you will appreciate more than the touch of a healing hand. Not many things will be more rewarding than knowing that you can help someone simply by laying your hands on them. The ultimate purpose of Dahnhak Hwal-Gong is to synchronize the minds of the giver and the receiver to bring about peace and joy. Hwal-Gong literally means to revive and to stimulate. It revitalizes the body and the mind; it is a "Shim-Bup", meaning "the way of the mind". Therefore, Hwal-Gong is more than just a technique. A Hwal-Gong giver must first prepare the right mindset toward the receiver. Extending a warm word with a comforting smile is also an essential aspect of Hwal-Gong.

The worst culprits in degenerating health are mindsets and lifestyles that go against life-supporting principles. If our minds wither in fear, our kidneys are weakened. If we sulk in depression, our lungs are weakened. If we burn in fury, our liver gets damaged. Aside from these internal organs, each branch of our nerves, veins, arteries; each fiber of our muscles; and every single cell in our body remembers and reacts to stress and emotional roller coasters. When these imbalanced states become chronic, 'Ki's' entry and exit points in our bodies get blocked, causing the meridians that connect our internal organs to malfunction. The root cause of many physical ailments start from here. Dahnhak Hwal-Gong is an effective method to rehabilitate balanced energy circulation by means of stimulating acupressure points and meridian channels.

It is said that ancient Korean sages comprehended the relationship between an illness and its root causes; they practiced preventing and remedying the root causes in their everyday lives. Dahnhak Hwal-Gong has adapted the wisdom of Korean ancestors to today's lifestyles. Our bodies are in their best state of health when they can be natural. The imbalance created by psychological stresses imposed upon the health of modern humans is caused by lifestyles that are disconnected from nature. This book is dedicated with our sincerest wish to help readers of this book recover their natural healthy state by using Dahnhak Hwal-Gong.

Dahn Healer School

Book **1**

Contents

Book ②

Preface

Hwal-Gong Classified by Symptoms

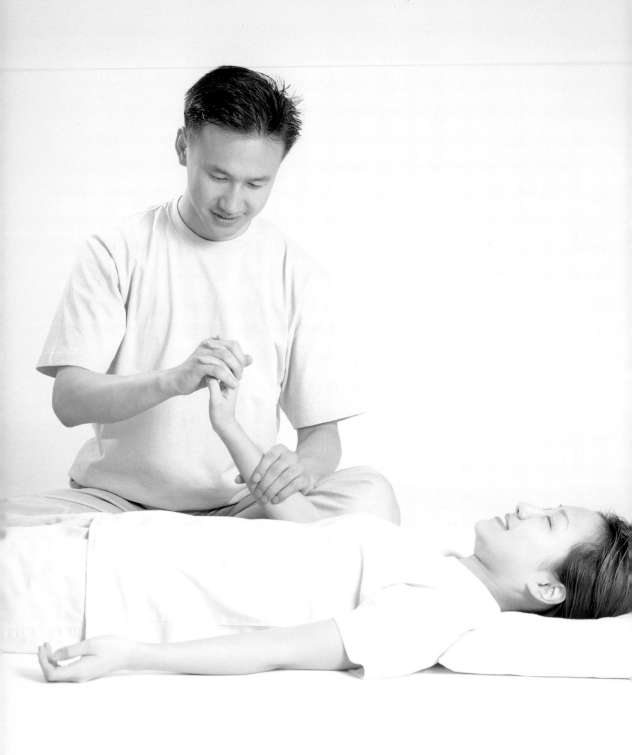

Chapter 1
What is Hwal-Gong?

1. Dahnhak Hwal-Gong is the Act of Giving Love

When our lower backs hurt, we automatically tap our backs. Needless to say, our hands go immediately to our stomachs when we have stomachaches. It is as though our hands have minds of their own. The acts of stroking, tapping, and touching the painful area are triggered by our instinctive reactions to heal ourselves. Touching and stroking our bodies is a natural healing and health method that is thousands of years old. Acupressure and massage are examples of such methods. Dahnhak Hwal-Gong has been developed by applying these methods to the modern Dahnhak principles. Dahnhak Hwal-Gong, in short, is the Act of Giving Love. In other words, it is an act of transmitting loving energy.

Basically, energy flows in our bodies and sustains our daily activities. Therefore, when 'Ki', the life energy, weakens, troubles arise in

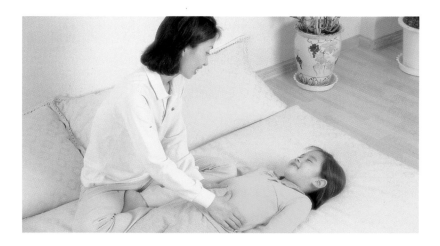

our body. When 'Ki' flow is blocked, our life energy does not circulate properly, and we become ill. By the same token, when 'Ki' flows excessively and overflows, it disrupts our energy balance, also causing us to be ill. Overworking, heavy drinking, overeating, excessive sex, and other excessive activities are the culprits that destroy energy balance. If we continue to live lives of excess, such lifestyles will naturally take a toll on our bodies. Illnesses are the body's warnings of when we break the rules of nature and abuse our bodies in daily life.

Hwal-Gong is not just a method used to treat disease but also a method to add vibrancy to life. In addition, Hwal-Gong heals the giver as well as the receiver, allowing for natural healing while healing others, too. Today, the global village is saturated with excessive amounts of competition and selfishness. People are obsessed with robbing and dominating others' energy. The Hwal-Gong method teaches that by helping others, you can help yourself. All who bestow Hwal-Gong to others in love and caring can feel their own bodies and minds become pure. This is a true act of love.

Hwal-In-Shim-Bang :
A book of strengthening the mind and body written by Toi-gye Lee, Whang (1501~1570) during the early Chosun Dynasty of Korea.
It includes ways to maintain and improve health and the life force. These drawings, by Toi-gye himself, are illustrations showing self-healing.

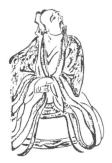
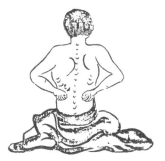
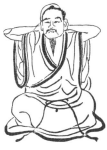

Hwal-Gong is a healing action using bare hands. It does not require the use of medicines or instruments. Mothers devotedly stroke their babies when their little ones get sick. Soon, the babies gaze up at their mothers with bright smiles on their faces as if nothing had ever bothered them. This is because their mothers' loving energies were transmitted through their hands. The most potent healing power in the world is the energy that comes from unconditional affection and devotion just as a mother might have for her baby. On the other hand, if someone stares at you in a towering rage, you may feel chills throughout your spine. As such, through our daily use of energy, we can exude the energy of love or the energy of hatred to our neighbors or colleagues. We choose to transmit certain types of energy for which we are responsible.

This is a mural found in a doctor's tomb in Sakara, Egypt that dates back 4,000 years. This indicates that they employed hands and feet in practicing reflexology to heal, as far back as in ancient Egypt.

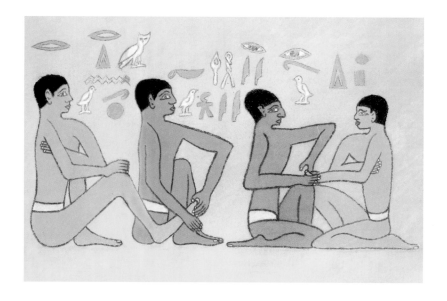

2. Seven Major Benefits of Dahnhak Hwal-Gong

1) Improving Blood Circulation

Hwal-Gong improves blood circulation, strengthens the walls of the blood vessels and alleviates the heart's workload. Enhancing blood circulation increases the oxygen and nutrients supplied to every part of the body. It also helps us recover from fatigue quickly.

2) Activating the Parasympathetic Response

When we get angry or excited, nerves or muscles become abnormally tense. Applying Hwal-Gong in such instances acts to placate the mind and re-balance the nerves and muscles.

3) Invigorating the Mind and Body

On the other hand, practicing Hwal-Gong when we feel exhausted and languid, creates a vitality that stimulates our bodies to restore normal function of our internal organs.

4) Realigning the Skeletal Frame

Most of us have unbalanced skeletal structure caused by our lifestyles. When we continue practicing Hwal-Gong over a long time, crooked bones and muscles return to their proper positions. Furthermore, applying Hwal-Gong to a sprain or bone injury after the swelling subsides, will prevent joints and tendons from setting in the injured condition.

5) Improving Functionality of Internal Organs

Hwal-Gong improves not only the skin and muscles, but also helps the internal organs function properly by controlling the energy flow within the body. It will improve digestion while alleviating constipation and diarrhea, as well as help the liver detoxify bood.

6) Improving Interpersonal Relations

Naturally, human contact brings people closer. In your spare time, if you frequently practice Hwal-Gong with your family members or colleagues, it will improve your interpersonal relationships.

7) Fostering Self-awareness and a Loving Heart

As we continue to render and receive Hwal-Gong, it allows us to step out of our shell and become aware of our surroundings. The heart will open, the ones who used to only be receivers will start to have desires to reciprocate by giving Hwal-Gong to others.

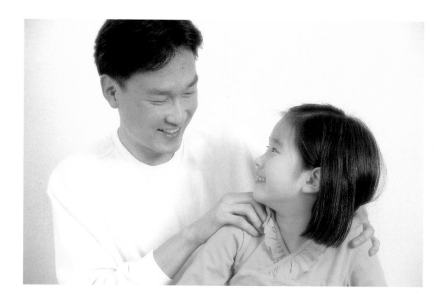

3. Three Principles of Dahnhak Hwal-Gong

1) Principle of Blood Circulation: Hwal-Hyul-Bup

By touching and stepping, Hwal-Gong improves blood circulation, and infuses our bodies with energy. Massaging can result in re-alignment of skeletal structure and enhancing blood circulation and energy flow.

2) Principle of Energy Circulation: Hwal-Ki-Bup

Practice this principle by gently laying a hand on someone else. This is a principle used to open up blocked acupressure points and meridian channels. By using our hands or by speaking, we can infuse another person with energy or remove stagnant energy from that person.

3) Principle of Calming : Hwal-Shim-Bup

You can practice Hwal-Gong by speaking. Words of confidence in the receiver's quick recovery will comfort the receiver's mind and benefit his/her physical health by transmitting positive energy. Hwal-Gong can also be practiced by eye contact. If the practitioner frowns while performing Hwal-Gong, the receiver will not feel comfortable receiving it. Energy can also be delivered through affectionate eye contact.

This drawing was discovered in the early 19th century in a book made of cut wood depicting people performing Hwal-Gong.

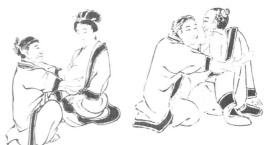

4. How to Touch

1) The Pressure Principle

There are three Pressure Principles in Dahnhak Hwal-Gong. They are Direct Pressure, Energy Pressure, and Mind Pressure. It is a rule in Hwal-Gong to apply direct pressure with energy and care at all times.

Direct-Pressure (Pressure)

Apply a moderate amount of pressure straight down on the target acupuncture points. In case of energy blockages and muscle spasms, a good amount of pressure is necessary to facilitate energy circulation and to relax the muscles.

Energy Pressure (Ki)

This pressure technique transmits energy. Energy is infused by applying a consistent amount of pressure for an extended period. While other massage techniques stimulate the body by use of pressure, Hwal-Gong stimulates the body by transmitting energy deep into the internal organs.

Mind Pressure (Synchronized Breathing)

The giver and the receiver of Hwal-Gong have to synchronize their breathing. Synchronized breathing means to inhale and exhale at the same time as the giver and the receiver attune their minds. This follows the same logic as a newborn chick breaking out of its shell: The breaking out of the shell is made easier as the mother hen pecks from outside and the chick pecks from within.

2) How to touch

Pressing with Thumbs

This is one of the most popular methods. Press downward with the face of your thumbs. As you practice this method, be careful not to use the tips of your thumbs, poking the receiver's body.

> ● NOTE
>
> The thumb's advantage over the other four fingers is that it can be used to accurately find and apply great pressure to a small point.

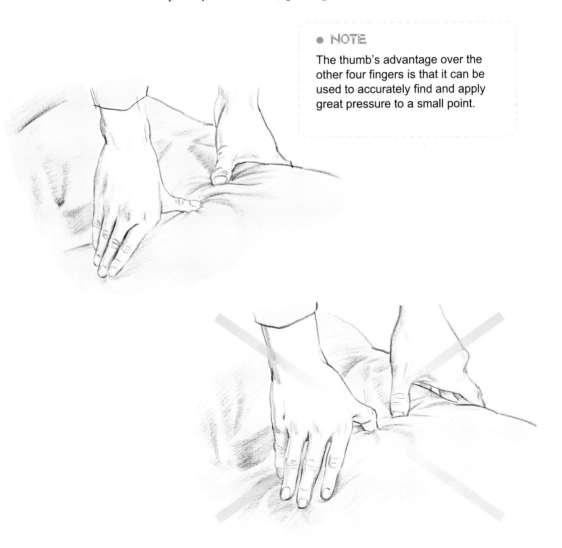

Pressing with Palms

This method, along with pressing with thumbs, is most frequently used. Use this method when the giver does not have to use much strength or cannot accurately locate a small point.

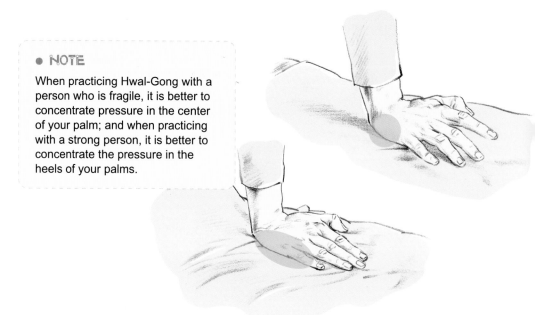

> ● NOTE
>
> When practicing Hwal-Gong with a person who is fragile, it is better to concentrate pressure in the center of your palm; and when practicing with a strong person, it is better to concentrate the pressure in the heels of your palms.

Pressing with Both Palms

The method of pressing with both palms is to press down with your hands placed one over the other. If you are right handed, your left hand should be on top.

> ● NOTE
>
> Press with consistent pressure, but not too hard.

Pressing with Both Thumbs

Press down with both thumbs one on top of the other. Press down on a precise spot. Use this method when you need to apply greater pressure than what one thumb can apply.

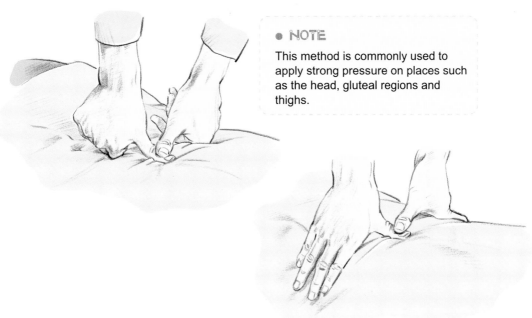

> **● NOTE**
>
> This method is commonly used to apply strong pressure on places such as the head, gluteal regions and thighs.

Massaging with the Hands

This method uses the five fingers. Forcefully grab an area as though kneading dough, and then release it.

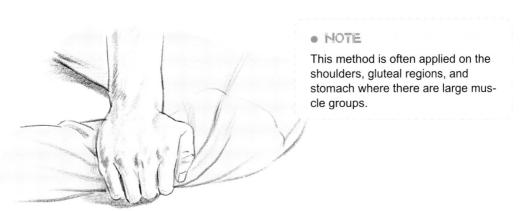

> **● NOTE**
>
> This method is often applied on the shoulders, gluteal regions, and stomach where there are large muscle groups.

Pressing down with Fists

To apply this method, you must make fists with both hands and then apply pressure by pressing down with your knuckles. It is important to apply even pressure with both fists.

> ● NOTE
>
> Gradually increase pressure for about five seconds. Be careful not to exert too much pressure.

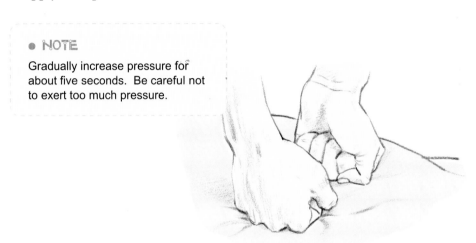

Pressing with the Elbows

Press down using the elbows. This method is used when you wish to apply pressure greater than the fists can provide. This method is not used very often.

> ● NOTE
>
> This method is used around the sacrum and in the lower gluteal area. Be careful not to use your elbow on the bone directly.

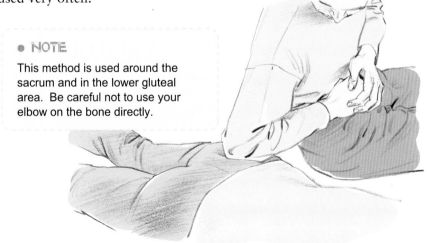

Pressing with Fingers

This method applies pressure using the palmar sides (fingerprinted sides) of the fingers excluding the thumb and the little finger. It is recommended to apply greater force with the third finger (middle finger) than with the other two.

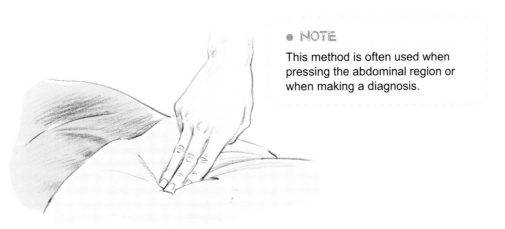

● NOTE

This method is often used when pressing the abdominal region or when making a diagnosis.

Shaking while Applying Pressure with Palms

This method involves shaking while applying pressure with both hands. This is easy to do, and is effective in improving blood circulation.

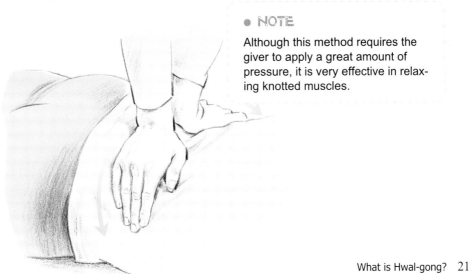

● NOTE

Although this method requires the giver to apply a great amount of pressure, it is very effective in relaxing knotted muscles.

Stepping with Feet

Walk on the receiver while he/she is lying down. This technique uses the full weight of the giver to easily apply pressure. Hwal-Gong exercises rarely use feet. To practice this method, the giver should be lightweight or a child.

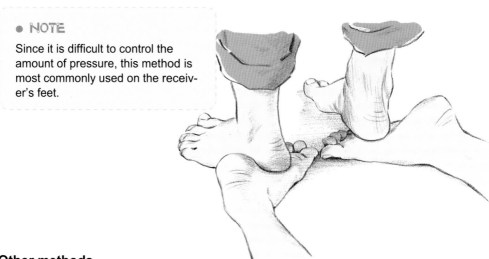

● NOTE

Since it is difficult to control the amount of pressure, this method is most commonly used on the receiver's feet.

Other methods

Rapping with fists, pulling with both hands, rubbing and unknotting, holding with palms, tapping with fingers, pushing, lifting and releasing with both hands, sending energy with hands, stroking with palms, shaking, pushing and rolling with hands.

Why are there so many different methods?

Do not be intimidated. When you get used to doing them, your hands will automatically know to which methods to use.

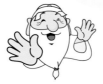

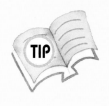

Aroma Hwal-Gong

A little bit of stress can give you an energy boost. However when stress exceeds the threshold, we get agitated, our mouths dry up, and our stomachs feel uncomfortable.

An effective way to relieve stress is to apply essential oils extracted from plants such as fruits, vegetables, or herbs on the body before practicing Hwal-Gong. Some aromatherapy can be done by direct application on the body, others by an inhalation, or infusion into bathwater.

To infuse it in bathwater, put 9~10 drops of oil into the bathwater, and stay in bath for about 15 minutes; or drop 2~3 drops of oil on a loufa scrub and rub it in with soap. If you are applying it on the body, dilute the essential oil in pure vegetable or body oil by a ratio of 2 to 98 or 3 to 97. Apply it all over the body. For direct inhalation, drop about 2 drops of the essential oil into a handkerchief or a facial tissue and inhale it deeply; or put 2 drops of an essential oil onto an aroma lamp to diffuse the scent into the air.

When you have difficulty sleeping due to stress, and feel tense, rub extracts (from rose, sandalwood, salvia, marjoram, or a cedar tree), into the body so that the therapeutic essence will penetrate and stimulate your body's pleasure centers.

In order to reduce stress, it is useful to massage your shoulders and neck. Concentrate on the back and then apply a little bit of Hwal-Gong around the face. In addition, it will be very helpful to foster good habits such as relaxed deep breathing and taking things easy in your daily life.

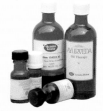

Scented oils are to be applied on the body during Hwal-Gong.

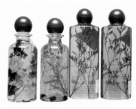

Essential oils are to be used for aromatherapy.

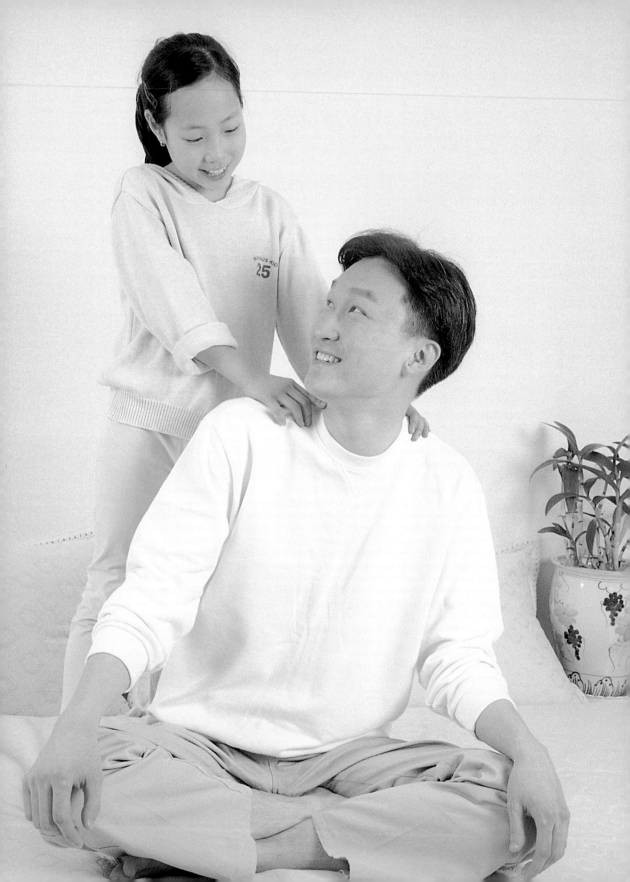

Chapter 2

Preparing for Hwal-Gong

1. Preparing for the Ideal Hwal-Gong Session

1) A Good Setting for Hwal-Gong

Bright colored sheets and covers

The area should be neat and clean. Prepare modest and simple tools to brighten up the hearts and minds of the givers and receivers.

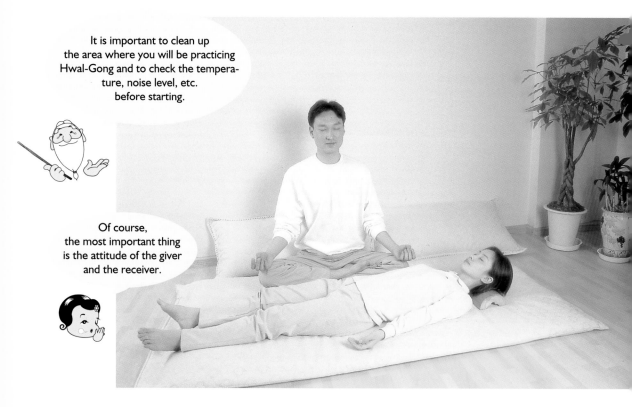

It is important to clean up the area where you will be practicing Hwal-Gong and to check the temperature, noise level, etc. before starting.

Of course, the most important thing is the attitude of the giver and the receiver.

Room temperature conducive to relaxing one's entire body

The temperature should be set at 20℃~25℃. This temperature is ideal for relaxation and allows one's energy to circulate well along muscle and acupressure paths.

Soft and tranquil lighting

Help the receiver of Hwal-Gong relax by adjusting the light to be a low and soothing level, yet refrain from making it too dim.

If you have prepared oils, music, scents, soft lighting, a mat and wood pillow (pillow made of empress tree) before starting Hwal-Gong, you are more than ready.

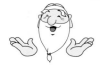

❶ Oil
It is good to prepare the oils to be used for a gentle Hwal-Gong session. Easily accessible body oils work, and essential oils used for aromatherapy work even better.

❷ Incense
Burning incense will clear and refresh your mind. Burning scented incense used for for specific symptoms, is especially effective. But it is best to ask your reciever first about using oils and incense because some people are sensitive to smell.

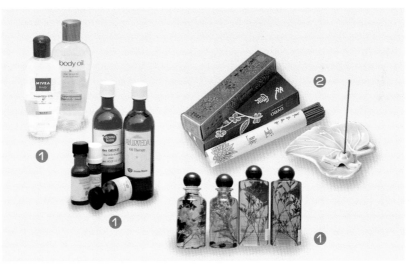

2) What a Hwal-Gong Giver should Keep in Mind

• Hwal-Gong is the act of giving love. Through the hands of the giver, the giver's unfiltered energy is sent to the receiver. The giver does this with utmost care and love toward the receiver.

• If the giver is not in a good condition, is in a bad mood, or is under stress, it is not recommended that he/she perform Hwal-Gong.

• Consider the receiver's age, personality, and the cause of illness. Make a note of the receiver's medical history, such as surgeries or other special circumstances.

• To maximize the benefits of Hwal-Gong, the giver should do hand exercises (See page 50.) before each session.

• Wash your hands thoroughly and keep nails trimmed (Long nails may cause pain to the receiver).

Shall we begin?
Let's go!
Let's go!

Hwal-Gong is not about boasting your own strength. Concentration and harmony of your mind and spirit are very important.

The most important thing of all is your loving heart. If you lack such caring emotion, the receiver will feel that something is amiss.

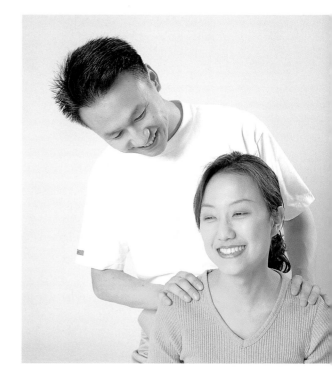

• Note that our body parts have reciprocal relationships. When someone has a headache, massaging their feet will allow the congested energy in the head to be released and flow toward the feet. For instance, when someone feels discomfort in the ventral (front) part of the body, has constipation or diarrhea, start by treating the dorsal (back) side of the body. When someone has a backache, start by treating the abdomen or the chest.

• Start treating a general area, and then gradually focus on the specific point of discomfort.

• Hwal-Gong should be done in a quiet and tranquil setting. However, sometimes, talking can help the receiver relax better.

3) What a Hwal-Gong Receiver should Keep in Mind.

• The receiver should use the restrooom before a session.

• Wear light and comfortable clothing, so the giver can palpate easily.

• Completely relax all your muscles and think happy thoughts. If you feel drowsy, just let yourself snooze.

• You should not receive Hwal-Gong when you are under the influence of alcohol.

• Avoid doing Hwal-Gong immediately after a meal. Wait at least 30-40 minutes after a meal before receiving Hwal-Gong.

• It is helpful to rest for about 10 minutes after a session. However, a prolonged lack of movement may cause your body to become too limp.

Relax your entire body. The receiver should take a "sleeping posture", also known as the "empty void posture". It means that you should completely relax your body as if it is merely dangling in space.

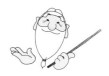

She falls asleep even before we start!

ZZZ...

4) Important Notes

• When the giver presses down on the receiver, the receiver should exhale through his/her mouth. When the giver releases his/her hand from the receiver, the receiver should inhale through his/her nose.

• When the giver and receiver are of opposite sex, the giver should be sensitive about making the receiver feel uncomfortable.

• Before exerting strong pressure on a point in the body, the giver must first softly touch the area. Just as you would do a sketch of something before etching a firm outline, perform a "Warm-up Hwal Gong" stroke.

Contraindications

• Do not treat patients of a systematic, contagious or infectious disease.

• Do not treat patients recovering from bone surgery.

• Do not treat patients with these symptoms or illnesses: cerebral hemorrhage, coma, diabetes with complications (such as gangrene), or other severe and chronic illnesses.

• When treating reproductive organs, do not treat the areas directly.

Let's start Warm-up Hwal-Gong.

5) Warm-up Hwal Gong

① Regulate your breathing. Close your eyes and spend about a minute to organize the Hwal-Gong procedures you are going to do. Imagine pure, bright energy flowing into your receiver.

② Place your palm on your receiver and pause for a moment to synchronize your breathing with the receiver's breathing.

③ Keep your hand on your receiver and softly rotate your hand in a clockwise direction. Feel your hand getting warmer.

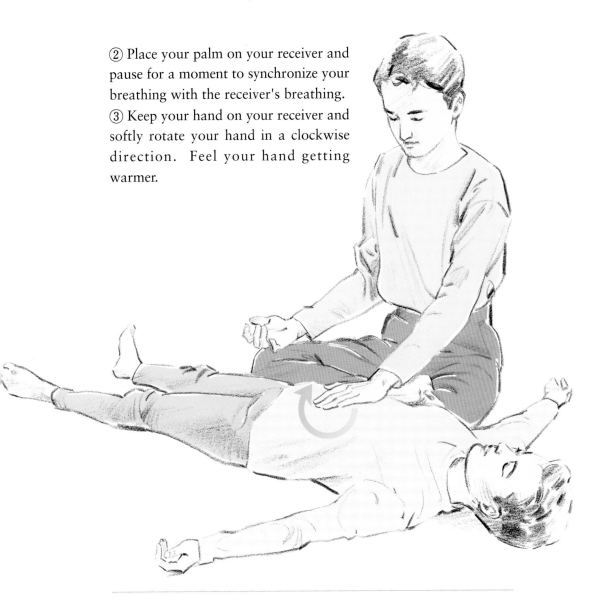

 When you do Warm-up Hwal Gong, always try to increase the pressure gradually as if you are melting some butter on the frying pan. If you put too much pressure from the beginning, the receiver will try to protect him/herself from the pressure by tightening the muscle and you will end up dealing with a body full of tension. Start rubbing the stomach with gentle movement.

2. Hwal-Gong 1, 2, 3...

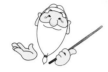

Once you are done with preparing for the Hwal-Gong session and Warm-up Hwal Gong, do the following.

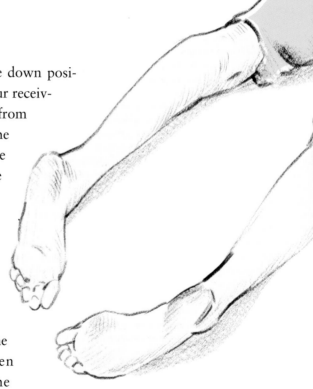

1) Prone Position

Begin with the receiver in a face down position. It is important to make your receiver feel that he/she can trust you from your first touch. If you begin the session with strong force, the receiver may subconsciously tense his/her body. Just as you would with a new pair of shoes, it may be necessary for the receiver's body to "break into" your touch. The giver has the responsibility to balance the receiver's body and treat it in a consistent manner. Work from the receiver's shoulders, and then release the back, the spine, the waist, and the gluteals to energize the body.

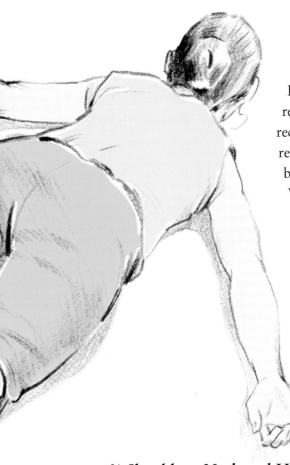

2) Back of the Legs (Thighs, Calves, Ankles, and Feet)

If tension in the upper body is relieved successfully, it means that the receiver trusted the giver, and therefore relaxed his/her entire body. You can begin to make your touch firmer. With precision and good body mechanics, even a robust male can step on a delicate female's foot to make her feet feel thoroughly released without inflicting pain. Go easy on the Achilles tendon and calves. However, tense thigh muscles may generally require stronger pressure before they become relaxed.

3) Shoulders, Neck and Head

People who perform mentally strenuous activities usually suffer tension in the above areas. When it is necessary to lift the receiver's face, the giver should have sure footing. When moving the receiver's head, do not use jerky or abrupt motions. Assist the receiver to shift his/her own head naturally and gradually. When doing so, the giver and receiver be able to feel their movements as one.

4) Face

One's face is a sensitive area. Therefore, it would be helpful to say, "I am now going to massage your face. You can stay relaxed."

Some people may have dry and sensitive skin. In this case, too much pressure may be irritating and unpleasant to the receiver. Ask your receiver if he/she has any allergies before using oils or creams. If your receiver is wearing make-up, ask her to wash it off before the session. If she does not wish to, just lightly tap the face and move on.

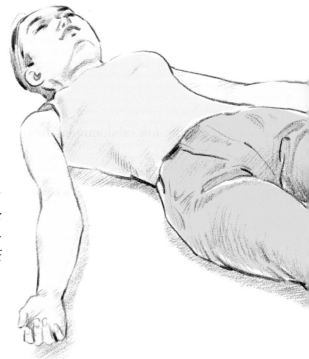

5) Arms and Hands (Palms)

If you feel tired or fatigued from giving Hwal-Gong at this point, have your receiver close his/her eyes and relax. You can use this time to do a light stretch. Arms and hands are very important areas for relieving fatigue. The transition from the head to the arms may not be so smooth. If the transition feels awkward, mend the gap by informing the receiver about the transition. The receiver will place more trust in the giver.

6) Chest and Abdomen

When treating a receiver of the opposite sex, make sure the receiver feels comfortable. It is especially important to control your breathing well, here. During chest Hwal-Gong, ask the receiver how he/she feels. He/She may say that he/she feels heat, chill, vibration, or a tingling sensation. However, if your receiver says he/she has no sensation in a certain area, remember everyone is different. During Dahn-jon (abdomindal area) Hwal-Gong, treat your receiver with your utmost care and dedication.

7) Front of Legs

When treating the front of the legs, avoid positioning yourself between the receiver's legs or assuming other sensitive position. It is necessary to use careful and natural body mechanics. It may be awkward at first, but with experience, you will become more and more comfortable, enabling your receiver to feel more comfortable too.

The elderly and children may be sensitive to even mild pressure. Ask an elderly receiver if he/she has arthritis or osteoporosis before treating his/her knee joints.

8) Sides of the Body

Make sure the receiver feels comfortable. Respect his/her body. Often, your hand positioning may feel awkward, so keep both of your hands placed on the receiver in a natural way and he/she will stay relaxed and comfortable.

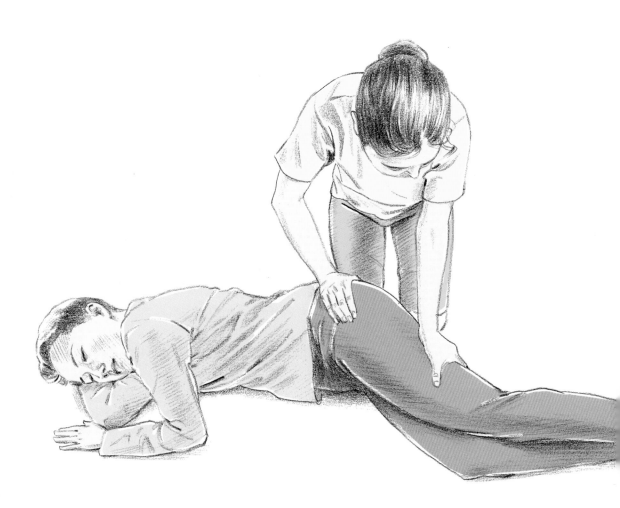

9) Sitting Position

It is recommended that the receiver be treated in this position prior to being treated in the prone position. There is a natural flow in first relieving the neck and shoulders and then working on the back of the body.

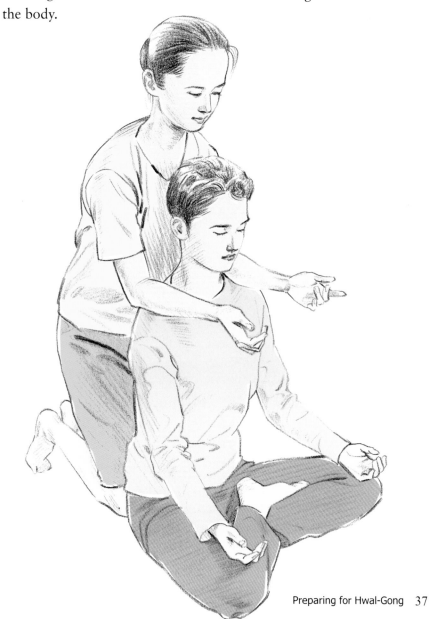

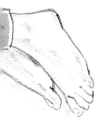

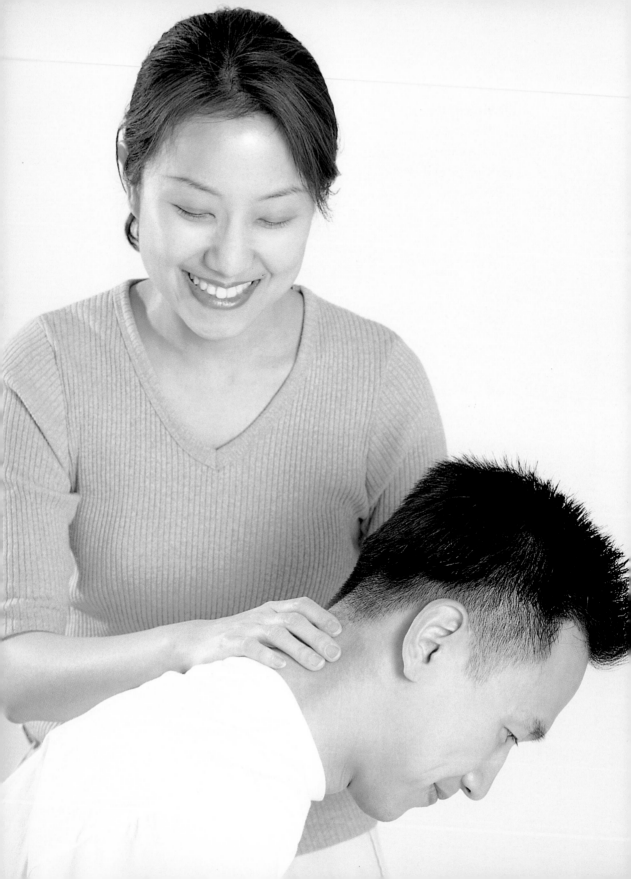

Chapter 3

Turning Your Hands into Healing Hands

1. Ki-energy and Healing Hands

All living things have internal energy. Ki exists undetected by the naked eye. From decades ago, the human mind's analytical and logical tendencies seeking explanations has instigated the development of a systematic and scientific method to study Ki-energy.

A Russian engineer named Semyon Kirlian invented the Kirlian camera, the most noteworthy example of such an endeavor in 1939. With a Kirlian camera, you can take a photograph of invisible Ki. When you take a picture of a leaf or a flower with this camera, you can see lights that are not visible to the naked eye. Interestingly enough, a fresh leaf, just taken from a tree, emanates a strong and clear light. However, if you take a picture of the same leaf after a couple of hours, the light emanating from the leaf is very weak; and eventually, once it has died, no light emanates at all from it.

Later, Professor Thelma Moss of UCLA captured the energy emanating from a patient with a Kirlian camera. It showed that after a Ki healing, the energy field increased. In addition, world-renowned universities and hospitals, including Columbia University and Harvard University, are developing treatments using Ki-energy and are conducting research on the subject. Recently, during the ninth Asian Pediatrics Conference held in Hong Kong, it was announced that touching a baby's body helps the baby's digestion, blood circulation, and respiratory function.

While the Western world is busy conducting scientific research to validate Ki-energy, people in the East are accustomed to using Ki-energy in their daily lives. They often apply their Ki-energy in intuitive and experimental ways through meditation or breathing exercises. For example, when children cry from stomachaches late at night, Asian mothers touch and stroke the baby's stomach, and recite, "Mommy's hands are healing hands." Then, miraculously, the baby stops crying and falls asleep. This type of folk remedy that every Korean may have experienced at one point in his or her life is an example of using Ki-energy in daily life.

Like in the aforementioned scenario, healing hands refer to transmitting the energy of love through the hands as a mother does stroking her baby's body. When you give Hwal-Gong, the giver's feeling is directly reflected in the giving action. Only when the giver's feeling is conveyed to care for and protect the receiver, can "Healing Hands" truly heal. Healing hands are not limited only to "Ki" masters or gurus who may know of special techniques. If there is genuine love, and the giver and the receiver can open their hearts and create harmony, the energy of love will naturally flow. Therefore, the Hwal-Gong giver who does not have love for the receiver cannot be said to have true "healing hands"; it deviates from the original intent of Hwal-Gong.

The principle of healing hands lies in faith. Healing hands do not require special techniques. The faith that stroking and touching a baby's stomach with your hands will cure an illness causes healing hands to emanate healing energy. Without such conviction, you cannot expect to achieve fundamental healing by merely and mechanically touching someone.

The left frame shows a photo of Ki-energy from a healthy person's hands taken by a Kirlian camera; the right frame shows a photo of the hands of a person who has an illness.

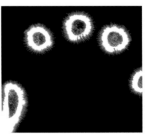 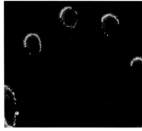

In Dahnhak, the principle of
healing hands is called "Shim-Ki-Hyul-Jung"
It means that if you touch another with
care and love, it will calm down
the receiver's mind. In turn,
when both minds are calm, our bodies' energy
and blood will also reach equilibrium.

Yes, that is true.
Just a hug from my mom makes
me feel better.
In fact, hugging with a loving heart
is the best Hwal-Gong.

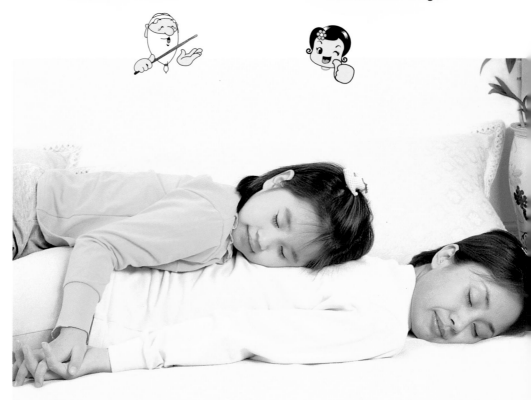

Babies who have received lots of
therapeutic touch develop much
stronger immune systems.

The best Hwal-Gong is
to embrace
a person with love.

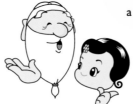

2. Warm-up Exercises to Turn Your Hands into Healing Hands

It is funny to think about a doctor with a cold treating a patient who has a cold. For the same reason, it is not desirable for the giver to give Hwal-Gong when his/her own body feels stiff. The giver is to sufficiently relax his/her own body prior to treating the receiver. Since it is an act of caring for someone else's body, having a caring attitude about one's own body is a natural prerequisite for a giver of Hwal-Gong. It would be even better if the giver would do the relaxation exercises with the receiver.

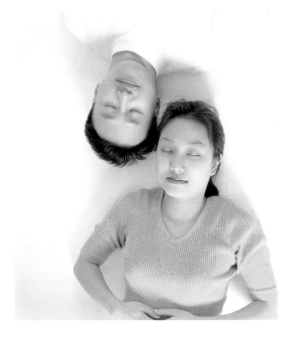

If the giver and the receiver both start in a relaxed state, it is as good as having completed half of the Hwal-Gong session.

❶ Make your entire body comfortable

1 Be in a comfortable sitting or standing position. As you deeply inhale, tuck in your neck as much as possible - like a turtle - and fold and bring your arms in against your chest. At the same time, bend your head forward.

2 Maintain this position for about 10 seconds and then exhale as you unbend and lower your arms and lift your neck. Repeat this several times.

❷ Relaxing your stomach (Making a circle)

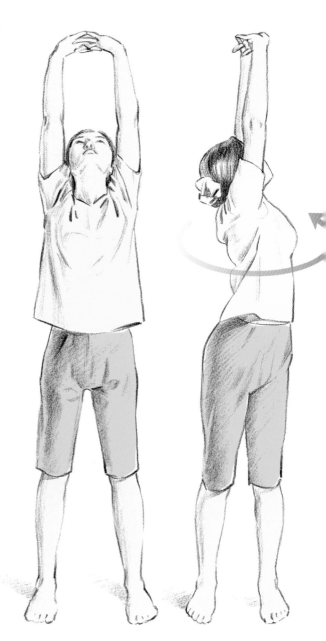

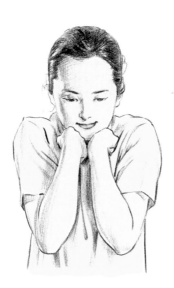

1   Stand with your legs shoulder width apart, clasping your hands together.

2   First, inhale, then lift your clasped hands up, and hold your breath.

3   Make a circle slowly turning your body clockwise with the torso deeply bent.

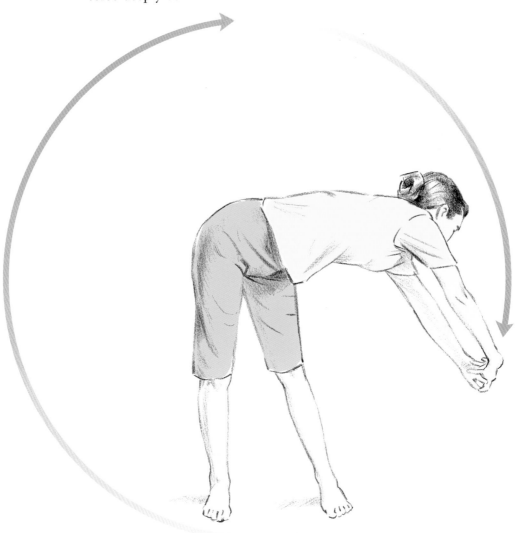

❸ Neck exercise

1 In a comfortable sitting or standing position, relax your neck by turning it left and right.

2 Bend your head to each side to let your ears touch your shoulders, and then bend it forward and backward.

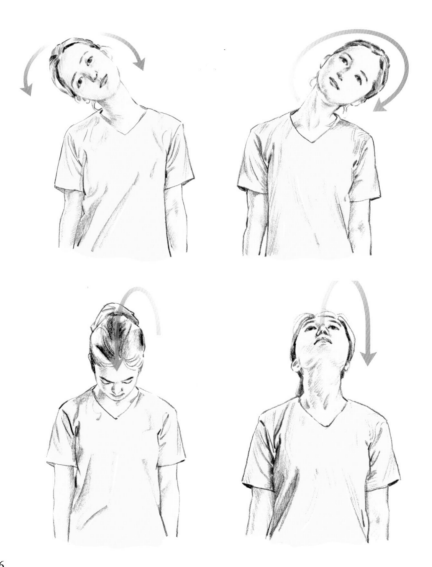

④ Arm twisting

1 Stretch out both of your arms with your fingers spread out. Spread your legs shoulder width apart.

2 As you inhale, twist your arms as much as possible with your little finger pointed upward. As you exhale, return to the original position.

3 Again, as you inhale, twist the arms as much as possible, this time with the thumb pointed downward. As you exhale, return to the original position.

4 Repeat several times.

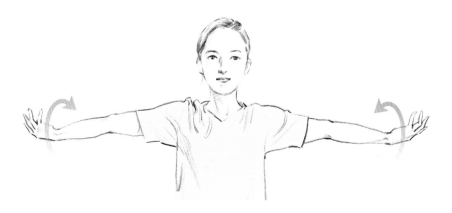

⑤ Stretching

1   In a sitting position, bring your legs together with the tips of your toes pointing straight up.

2   In this position, clasp both of your hands.

3   While inhaling, hold the tips of your toes with your clasped hands.

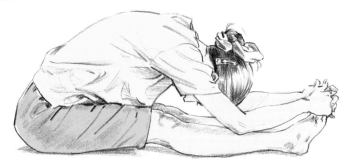

4   While exhaling, return to the starting position, and spread out your legs as widely as possible.

5   Again, while inhaling, bend your upper body (facing your left knee) so that your clasped hands can touch your left ankle.

6   While exhaling, return to the starting position. Do the same stretch in the other direction.

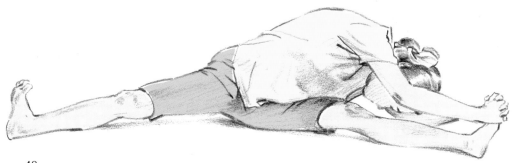

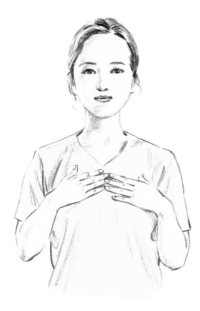

⑥ Tapping the chest

1 While standing, spread your legs shoulder width apart, and tap your chest with both of your palms.

2 It is good to tap the whole body in the same manner as well.

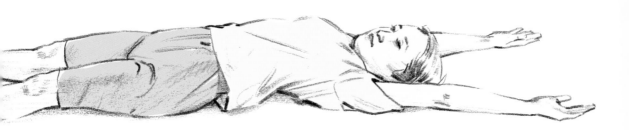

⑦ Stretching out the body

Stretch the whole body with arms stretched up all the way. Afterwards, meditate while focusing on your Dahn-jon (abdominal area). Finish up by breathing deeply a couple of times with your arms open wide.

3. Hand Exercises to Turn your Hands into Healing Hands

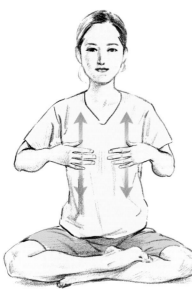

① Shake hands

While sitting, lift up your hands to the level of your solar plexus. Relax your hands and shake them very fast. Feel the increasing weight and warmth in your hands.

② Clap your hands

Stretch open your palms, focus on your hands, and clap 30 times. Now, relax all muscles in your hands while continuing to focus your thoughts on them.

③ Rub your hands

Your hands are hot after the clapping session. More sensitized healers may also feel a sense of relief in the chest. Now, inhale and hold your breath for about 10-20 seconds while vigorously rubbing the hands.

❹ Release the finger joints

Open your hands and exercise your finger joints. It is also good to massage the joints.

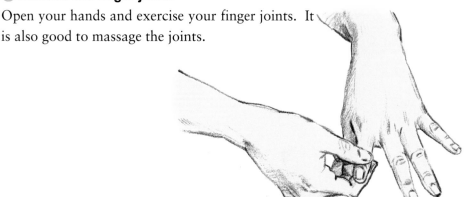

❺ Fist exercise

Make a fist and release. You may feel heat, heaviness, or something enveloping your hands. If you do not sense anything, keep concentrating. If you still do not feel anything, rub your hands and try again. Some people are more sensitized than others are. This is not a serious matter. The important thing is to always think of the person to whom you will be giving Hwal-Gong and relax your fists accordingly.

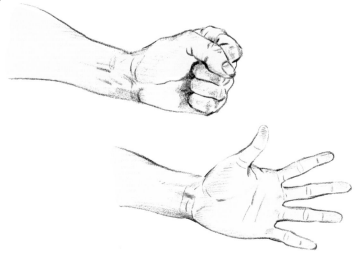

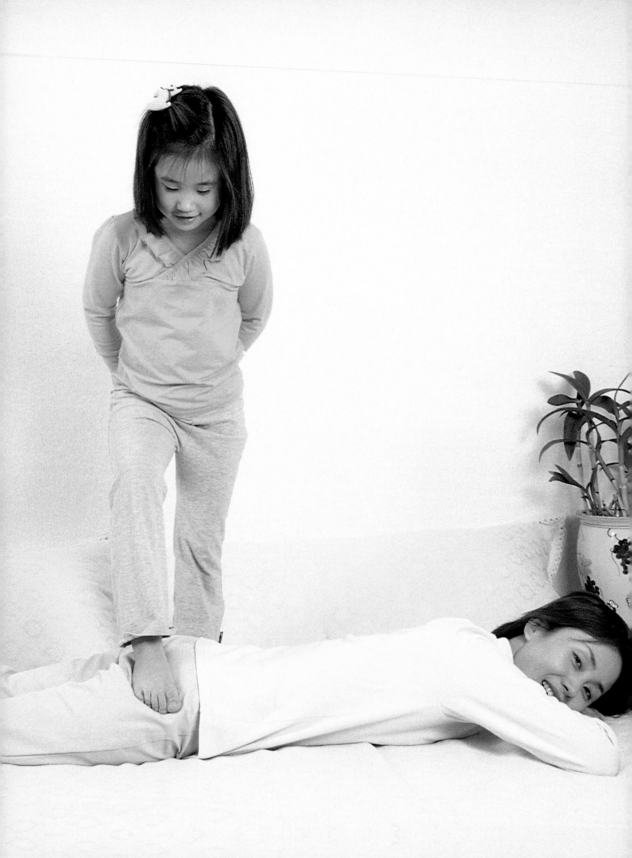

Chapter 4

Back Side of the Torso and Hips

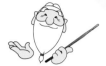

Nerves are spread throughout
the body from the top of the head to
the tips of your toes, and all of the major
nerves pass through the
spinal cord inside the spine.
Well, shall we start from the back?

Of the many features on the dorsal surface of our bodies, our back the most broadly shaped, and therefore are the strongest areas. The back's spinal column consists of the neck's 7 cervical bones, the torso's 12 thoracic vertebrae, the waist's 5 lumbar bones, one sacral bone, and one tailbone in the gluteal region. Similar to a spider web, our nervous system spreads out from the spine (or vertebrae) and spreads throughout our bodies.

The meridian channels that flow throughout our bodies run like expressways over our arms and legs. The most notable channels that flow on the dorsal surface are the Dok-maek (Governor Meridian) and the Urinary Bladder Meridian. The Urinary Bladder Meridian which governs "water" energy, maintains and sustains our bodies. Too much fatigue or excessive sexual activities may cause an imbalance in the Urinary Bladder Meridian.

A good Hwal-Gong session on the back alone can improve the receiver's condition. In addition, in case of stomach discomfort, it is recommended to begin by treating the back and gradually moving toward the front of the body.

When giving Hwal-Gong on someone's back, have the receiver lie face down. Depending on the Hwal-Gong guidelines, have the receive face forward or on the side of thier face.

So, that's
why it feels
so good to have
my back
scratched!

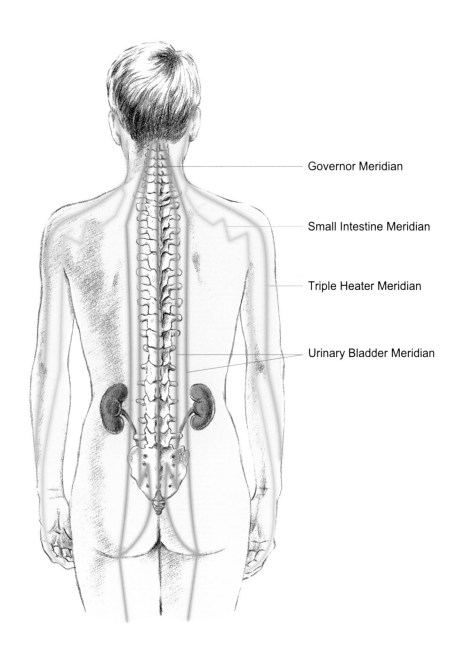

Governor Meridian

Small Intestine Meridian

Triple Heater Meridian

Urinary Bladder Meridian

Meridians flowing on the back of the body

There is a natural principle called Su-Seung-Hwa-Gang. It describes water energy of the kidneys riding upward along the back of the body, and fire energy flowing on the anterior part of the body downward toward the abdomen. When Su-Seung-Hwa-Gang is working properly, a person's head feels cool and the abdomen warm. Unfortunately, many people today have hot heads and cold abdomens instead. Their energy is concentrated in their heads and circulates poorly. This state is described as "Sang-Ki" or "Upset Energy." When you are "upset" your head feels cloudy or hot, and your abdomen or feet feel cold. This condition is also accompanied by symptoms of diarrhea.

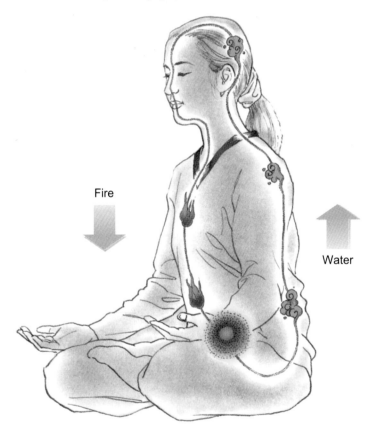

Fire

Water

State of Su-Seung-Hwa-Gang

1. Relaxing the Shoulder Muscles

Hwal-Gong Techniques

Massaging with hands, pressing with thumbs

Benefits

Helps relieve hypertension, neck tension, and frozen shoulders.

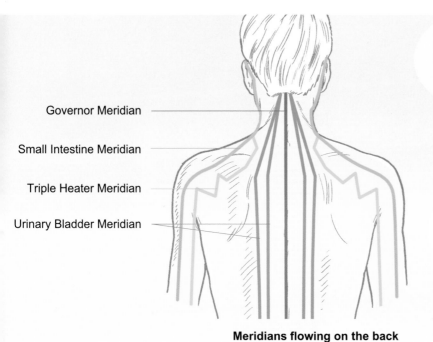

Governor Meridian

Small Intestine Meridian

Triple Heater Meridian

Urinary Bladder Meridian

Meridians flowing on the back

Before you work on someone else's back and spine, relax by releasing the tension in your shoulders first.

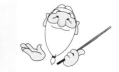

Ah ha! Relaxing the shoulders is the key to receiving good Hwal-Gong.

1 Have the receiver lie on his/her stomach, facing forward (chin on the floor). If this is uncomfortable, he/she may face sideways.

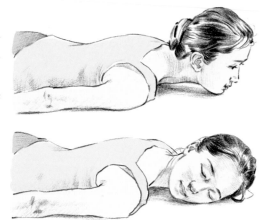

2 Sit by the receiver's side. Rub your hands and make them hot. Grasp the receiver's upper trapezius muscles with pressure, and then release. Repeat.

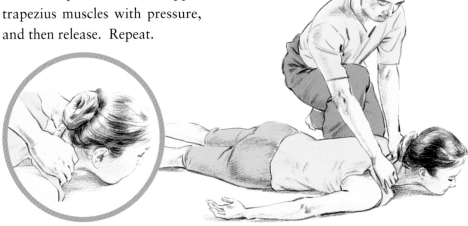

3 After sufficiently relieving the receiver's shoulder tension, press your thumbs along the receiver's shoulders. Move from the medial to the lateral points.

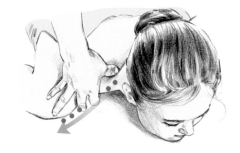

2. Relaxing the Shoulder Blades

Hwal-Gong Techniques

Massaging with hands, pressing with thumbs

Benefits

Helps relieve constipation, indigestion, colon and stomach dysfunctions, bronchitis, pneumonia, shoulder pain, and frozen shoulders.

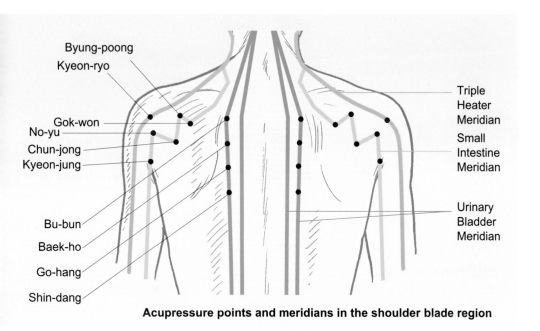

Acupressure points and meridians in the shoulder blade region

Don't forget to begin with
Warm-up Hwal Gong.
Remember, from page 31
You can build rapport with
the receiver through Warm-up
Hwal Gong.

All that I can remember is
the makeup analogy…

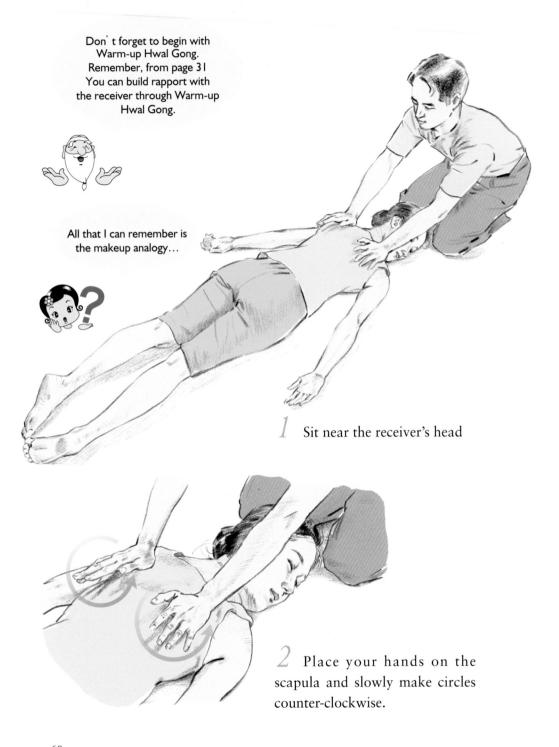

1 Sit near the receiver's head

2 Place your hands on the
scapula and slowly make circles
counter-clockwise.

3   Sit on the left side of the receiver.

4   Place the receiver's right hand (palm up) on his/her back and hold the receiver's right shoulder joint.

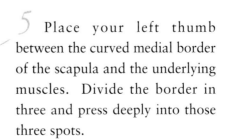

5   Place your left thumb between the curved medial border of the scapula and the underlying muscles. Divide the border in three and press deeply into those three spots.

6 Keep your thumb on the scapula border and bring the receiver's shoulder toward you. Hold for 5 seconds and release. Lift the shoulder enough so a part of the receiver's chest is lifted also, and press inward with your thumb at the same time.

7 Have the receiver exhale during the lift and inhale upon the release.

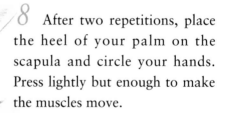

8 After two repetitions, place the heel of your palm on the scapula and circle your hands. Press lightly but enough to make the muscles move.

The scapula is a region where many meridian channels flow and is susceptible to blockage. Effectively releasing just the scapula region can invigorate the entire body.

3. Relaxing the Back by Rubbing and Pressing

Hwal-Gong Techniques

Pressing with both palms

Benefits

Helps relieve the Urinary Bladder Meridian to recover the kidneys' ability to elevate the body's water energy and increase the entire body's energy. It is also good for relieving fatigue and helps treat stomach problems.

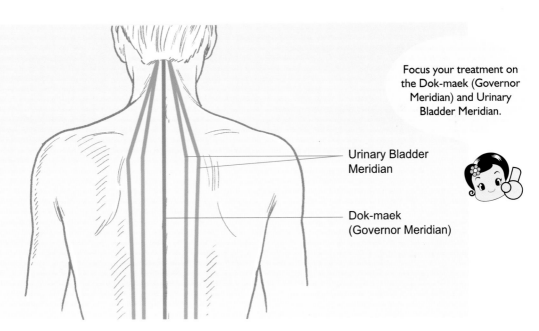

Focus your treatment on the Dok-maek (Governor Meridian) and Urinary Bladder Meridian.

Urinary Bladder Meridian

Dok-maek (Governor Meridian)

More important than pressing
the specific acupressure points is
the intention and devotion to treating
the entire back... Start with
Warm-up Hwal Gong.

1 Place your right palm on the
receiver's back. Put your left
hand over it. Position your hands
perpendicularly to each other so
that your right fingers are pointing toward the receiver's head.

2 Gradually press downward
and let the receiver exhale. Ask
your receiver to hold his/her
breath and circle your hands to
release muscle tension in the
receiver's back.

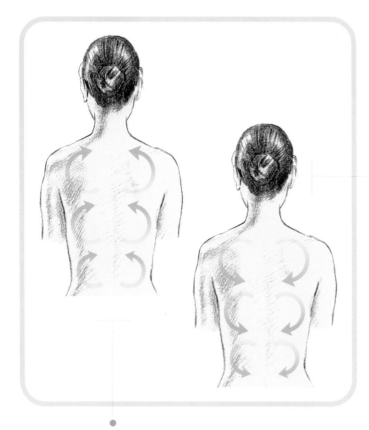

**When the receiver's body
is hypertonic (too tense)**
Apply strong pressure on
your bottom hand as well
as your top hand and make
downward circles toward
the hips when massaging.

When the receiver's body is hypotonic (too weak)
Use the bottom hand as support and apply pressure
with your top hand. Massage in an upward, circular
motion toward his/her head.

3 To finish off, rub
the entire back in a cir-
cular motion.

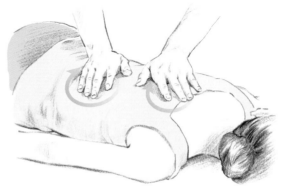

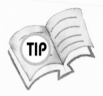

Hwal-Gong for the Elderly

The elderly tend to have weak bones and muscles, and may tend to suffer from indigestion, diarrhea, and constipation. They may have dulled sensation throughout their bodies; they may be experiencing loss of appetite; and they may be susceptible to depression. In general, an elderly person has decreased Ki-energy, therefore, a toning Hwal-Gong is recommended. In addition, because an elderly person's Won-Ki (inherited strength or energy) has depleted by this point, it is good to help him/her to gain energy from outside sources by strengthening his/her digestive system. Address his/her frequent location of pain. Most importantly, have love and respect for the elderly.

Contraindications when Giving Hwal-Gong to the elderly

- When massaging an elderly person's knees or other joints, focus on his/her acupressure points as you apply pressure.
- Keep up a conversation with the receiver to get feedback. This also allows pent up, negative emotions to be released.
- Take precautions when working around weak bones. Take special care during "alignment" Hwal-Gong when you have your elderly receiver in a prone position

4. Shaking while Pressing the Lower Back

Hwal-Gong Technique

Pressing with palms

Benefits

Helps relieve tension in the legs, reduces lower back pain, and improves problems in the reproductive system by strengthening the Urinary Bladder Meridian. Strengthening the Urinary Bladder Meridian can also alleviate symptoms of sciatica, menstrual cramps, leukorrhea, eczema, and fatigue.

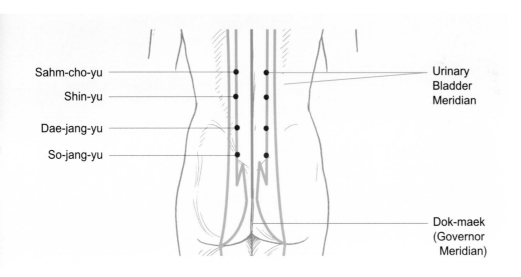

Sahm-cho-yu

Shin-yu

Dae-jang-yu

So-jang-yu

Urinary Bladder Meridian

Dok-maek (Governor Meridian)

1 Have the receiver overlap his/her hands and place them below the navel. If this is uncomfortable, a different, natural position is okay.

2 Wrap your hands around the receiver's waist by having the heels of your palm touch each other (over the lumbar vertebrae), and fingers pointing laterally.

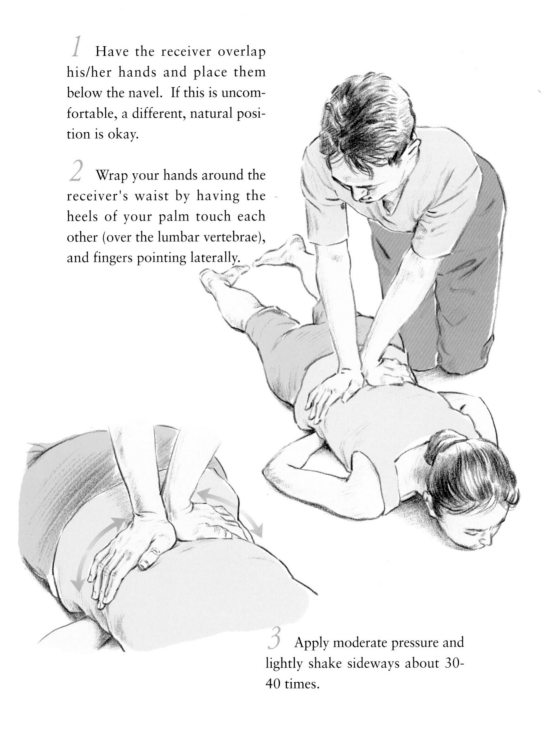

3 Apply moderate pressure and lightly shake sideways about 30-40 times.

5. Pressing and Rocking the Gluteal Region

Hwal-Gong Technique

Pressing with palms

Benefits

This stimulates the Urinary Bladder Meridian flowing toward the lower body and is good for relieving fatigue and strengthening the reproductive system. This can also stimulate the large intestine, which will alleviate constipation and diarrhea. This is also helpful in correcting irregular menstruation and sciatica.

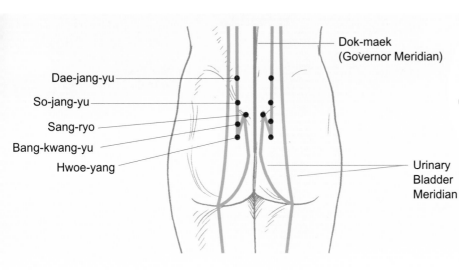

Dae-jang-yu

So-jang-yu

Sang-ryo

Bang-kwang-yu

Hwoe-yang

Dok-maek
(Governor Meridian)

Urinary
Bladder
Meridian

Dok-maek and
Urinary Bladder
Meridian are released.
Depending on individual conditions, you may
focus more on one of
the two meridians.

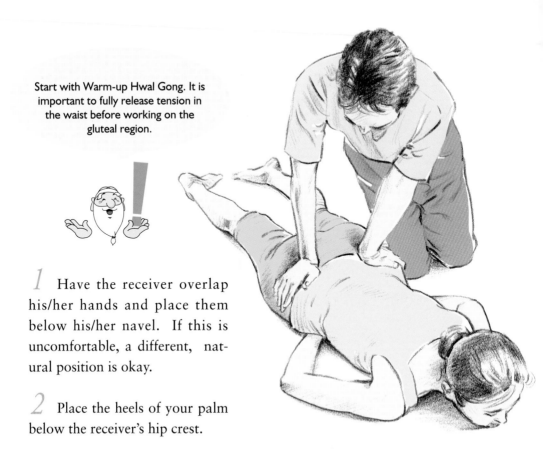

Start with Warm-up Hwal Gong. It is important to fully release tension in the waist before working on the gluteal region.

1 Have the receiver overlap his/her hands and place them below his/her navel. If this is uncomfortable, a different, natural position is okay.

2 Place the heels of your palm below the receiver's hip crest.

3 Alternate pressures to and from each hand. Press and shake, gently.

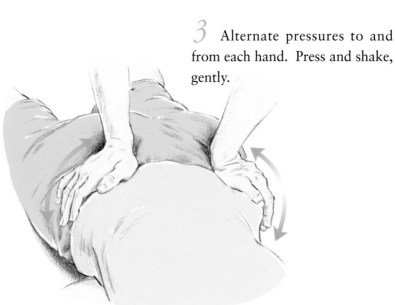

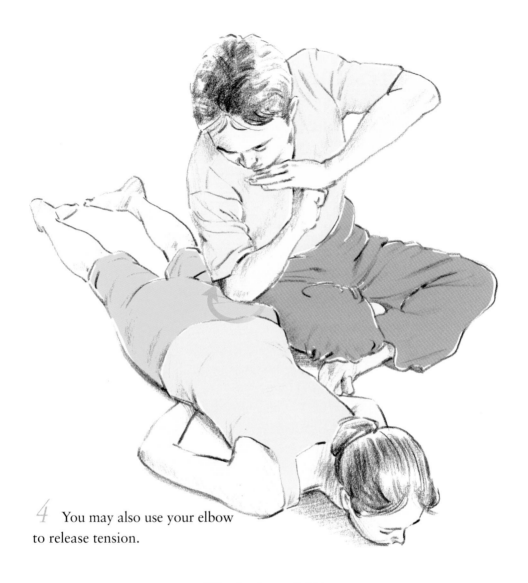

4 You may also use your elbow
to release tension.

If the giver is a small child
or is light-weight,
the giver can use the foot stepping
method on the receiver's feet.

6. Pressing the Spine

Hwal-Gong Technique

Pressing with thumbs

Benefits

The basic Hwal-Gong principle says to start working on the back when treating a stomachache or other abdominal problems. Treating the back can help relieve gastrospasms, abdominal cramps, sciatica, diarrhea, and constipation. It is also good for treating urinary system disorders and diabetes.

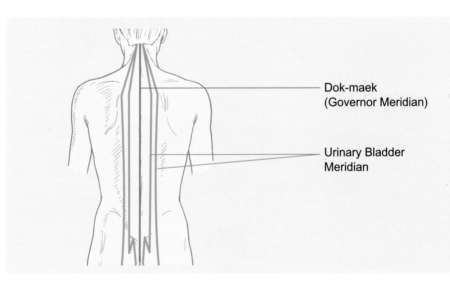

Dok-maek
(Governor Meridian)

Urinary Bladder
Meridian

1 After relaxing the shoulder muscles, press your thumbs along spinal line 1 and 2 (see p.74).

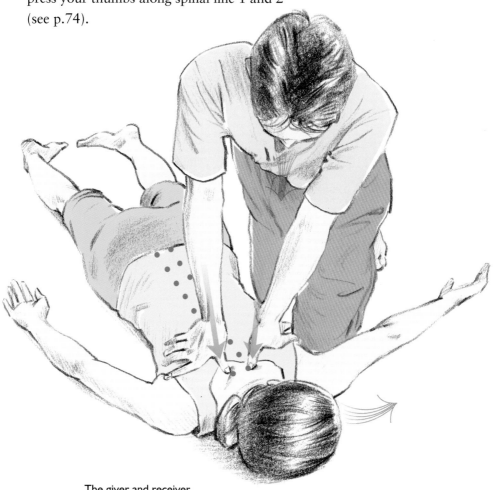

The giver and receiver should synchronize their breathing.

When the receiver exhales, the giver should exhale also.

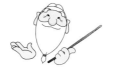

_1_ First, start from the thoracic vertebra (the most prominent protrusion in the spine) and press along the lines right next to the spinous processes. Press every 1-2 inches. This is spinal line 1. When the giver presses down, the receiver should exhale.

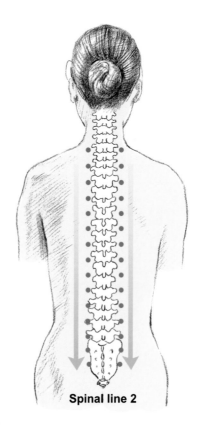

Spinal line 2

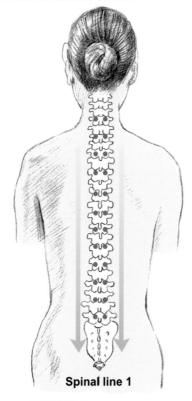

Spinal line 1

_2_ In the same way you pressed along spinal line 1, press along spinal line 2. Start around the transverse processes of T1 down to the sacrum.) As the receiver exhales, press down while pushing in an upward direction. Apply pressure at a point where you cannot push upward any further.

Be careful not to press too hard around the lumbar region. The bones in the lumbar region can be easily dislocated. So, apply lighter pressure.

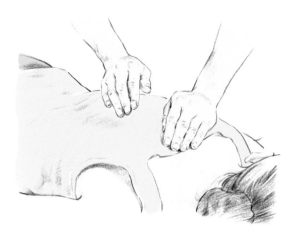

Finishing up Hwal-Gong on the back of the body

3 Finally, cup your hands and tap the receiver's back from top to bottom. Smooth his/her back with your palms. You can omit the tapping if the receiver has weak muscles.

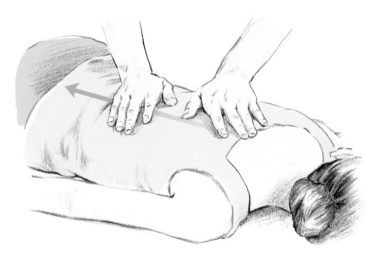

Smoothing down to finish up reconnects the meridian channels and further expels stagnant energy.

And now, we are finished with the back!

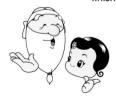

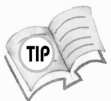

Structure of the Spine

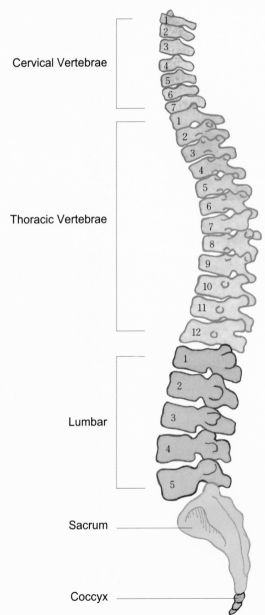

Cervical Vertebrae

Thoracic Vertebrae

Lumbar

Sacrum

Coccyx

Dysfunctions Caused by Problems in Each Vertebra

- Cervical Vertebrae 1-3   [Ah-moon]   : causes language problems, vision problems, pain and heaviness in the occipital region
- Cervical Vertebrae 3-7   [Chun-ju]   : headaches, pain behind the head, poor vision, deafness, frozen shoulders.

- Thoracic Vertebrae 1   [Dae-chu]   : neuralgia, hemorrhoids, asthma, hives, pneumonia, muscle pains in the upper extremities

- Thoracic Vertebrae 2   [Poong-moon]   : cold, insomnia, motion sickness, anemia
- Thoracic Vertebrae 3   [Pae-yu]   : coughing, asthma, hives, tight shoulders
- Thoracic Vertebrae 4   [Kwol-yeum-yu]   : leukorrhea, heart problems, memory loss, anxiety
- Thoracic Vertebrae 5   [Shin-do]   : forgetfulness, angina, anxiety, heart problems
- Thoracic Vertebrae 6   [Young-dae]   : asthma, anxiety, bronchitis, angina
- Thoracic Vertebrae 7   [Ji-yang]   : headaches, migraines, insomnia, dyspepsia, gastric ptosis
- Thoracic Vertebrae 8   [Gyuk-yu]   : insomnia, gastro spasm, pain in underarms, stomachaches
- Thoracic Vertebrae 9   [Gahn-yu]   : insomnia, nausea, gastric problems, hives, asthma, foot problems
- Thoracic Vertebrae 10   [Dahm-yu]   : gastric problems and chronic gall bladder infection
- Thoracic Vertebrae 11   [Be-yu]   : chronic gastric problems, diabetes, anemia, loss of appetite, skin disorder
- Thoracic Vertebrae 12   [We-yu]   : chronic pain, abdominal pain, skin disorder

- Lumbar 1   [Sahm-cho-yu]   : loss of vitality, abdominal pain, hemorrhoids, skin disorder
- Lumbar 2, 3   [Myung-moon]   : abdominal pain, menstrual irregularity, tinnitus
- Lumbar 4   [Dae-jang-yu]   : abdominal pain, diverticulitis, constipation, diarrhea, hives, neuralgia
- Lumbar 5   [Yo-yang-gwan]   : bladder infection, leukorrhea, abdominal pain, sciatica

- Sacrum, upper   [So-jang-yu]   : dysfunction in reproductive organs, lower abdominal pain, swelling of feet
- Sacrum, lower   [Bang-gwang-yu]   : bladder infection, cervical cancer, problems with ovaries

* Words in brackets refer to the names of acupressure points in the corresponding spinal area.

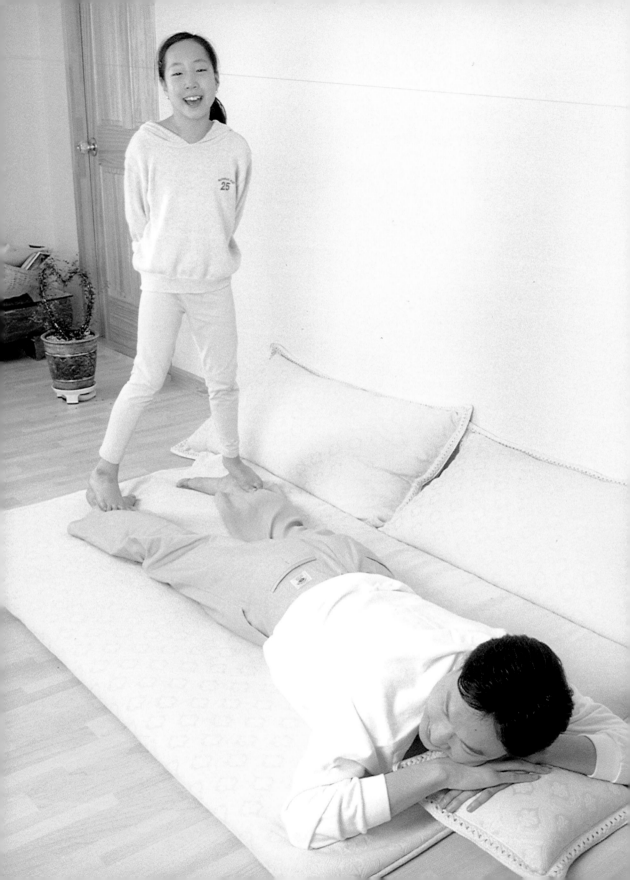

Chapter 5

Back of the Legs

Our legs are the main supports for our bodies, and so it's easy for them to become tired. A good leg Hwal-Gong will chase away fatigue.

We walk with all our weight placed on our legs. The area between the hip joints and the thighs is supported by a set of massive muscles. The weight-bearing knee joints control the front and back movements. Our legs and feet are positioned inward relative to the rest of body. This makes our lower backs and knees susceptible to fatigue and pain. Frequent walks as well as maintaining good energy circulation of meridians from the waist to the feet are recommended. In the center of the backside of the legs is the Kidney Meridian; and to the side in the back is the Urinary Bladder Meridian. These meridian channels are related to the kidneys; they carry "water" energy and protect the kidneys. Water is the source of life. No living creature can survive without it. Hence, if your kidneys' water energy is depleted you may be easily fatigued and become listless.

Just like the back torso, the posterior sides of the legs have a "Yang" characteristic. The legs are made of well-toned, massive muscles, and have abundant adipose tissues. The leg area requires more pressure for releasing energy blockages. Heels of palms are frequently used, and feet can be used on these areas, as well.

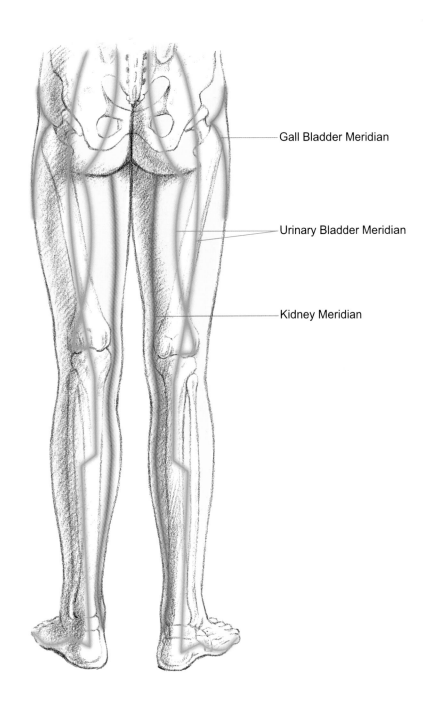

Gall Bladder Meridian

Urinary Bladder Meridian

Kidney Meridian

1. Pressing the Soles

Hwal-Gong Techniques

Stepping with feet, tapping with fists

Benefits

Plantar surfaces of the feet are where numerous meridian channels and acupressure points are concentrated. Therefore, treating the feet can treat all kinds of ailments. This technique is especially effective for relieving fatigue.

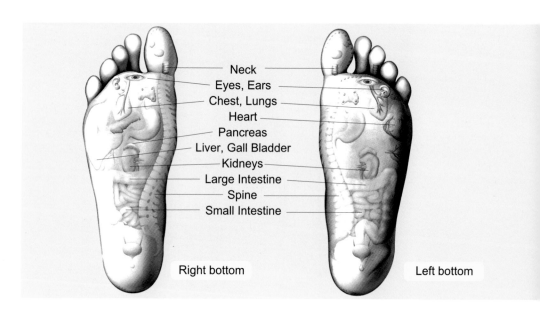

Neck
Eyes, Ears
Chest, Lungs
Heart
Pancreas
Liver, Gall Bladder
Kidneys
Large Intestine
Spine
Small Intestine

Right bottom

Left bottom

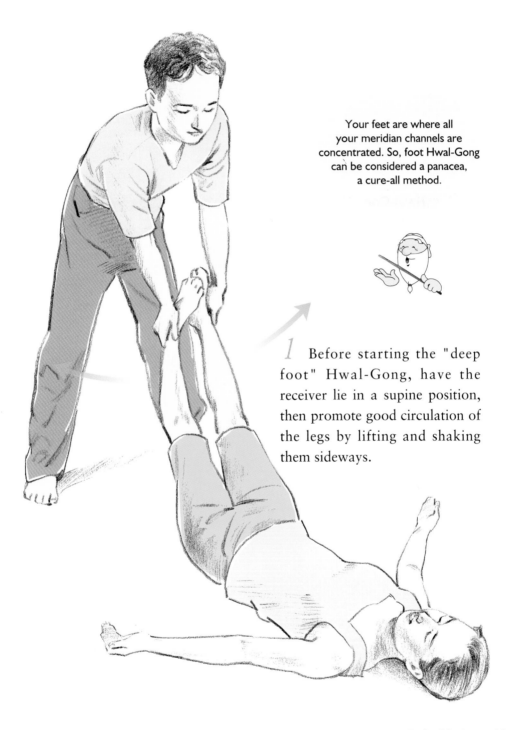

Your feet are where all
your meridian channels are
concentrated. So, foot Hwal-Gong
can be considered a panacea,
a cure-all method.

1 Before starting the "deep
foot" Hwal-Gong, have the
receiver lie in a supine position,
then promote good circulation of
the legs by lifting and shaking
them sideways.

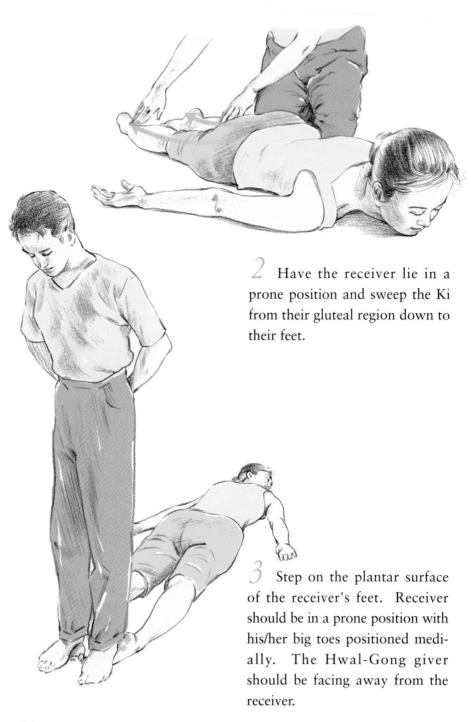

2 Have the receiver lie in a prone position and sweep the Ki from their gluteal region down to their feet.

3 Step on the plantar surface of the receiver's feet. Receiver should be in a prone position with his/her big toes positioned medially. The Hwal-Gong giver should be facing away from the receiver.

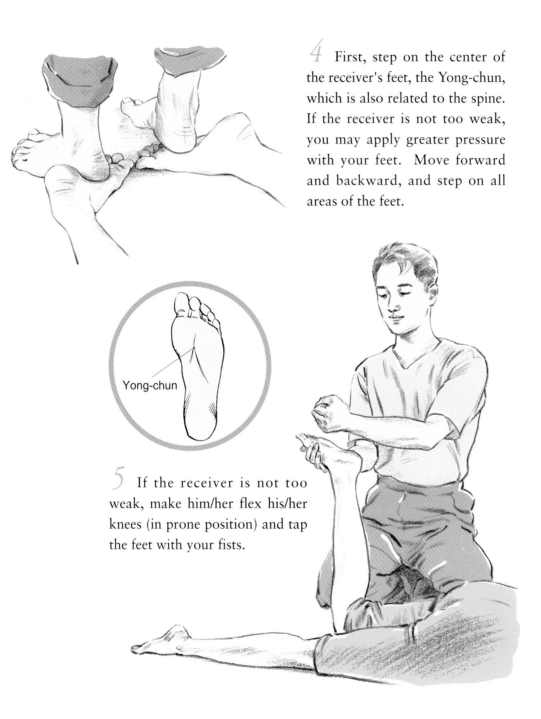

4 First, step on the center of the receiver's feet, the Yong-chun, which is also related to the spine. If the receiver is not too weak, you may apply greater pressure with your feet. Move forward and backward, and step on all areas of the feet.

Yong-chun

5 If the receiver is not too weak, make him/her flex his/her knees (in prone position) and tap the feet with your fists.

2. Shaking the Ankles

Hwal-Gong Technique

Compressing while shaking

Benefits

Strengthens the vertebrae, relieves the Urinary Bladder Meridian, helps your urination become normal and relieves menstrual cramps. It is also good for treating a stiff neck.

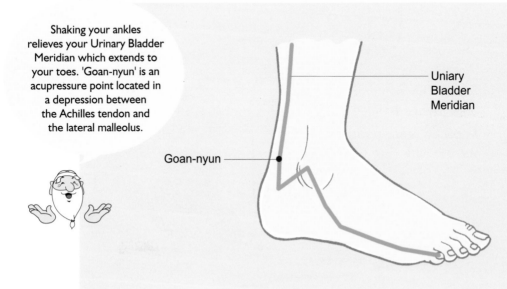

Shaking your ankles relieves your Urinary Bladder Meridian which extends to your toes. 'Goan-nyun' is an acupressure point located in a depression between the Achilles tendon and the lateral malleolus.

Uniary Bladder Meridian

Goan-nyun

Be careful not to press
the Achilles tendon
too hard.

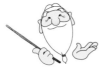

1 Kneel by the receiver's feet. Gently press the receiver's Achilles tendon, and shake it.

2 Shake the left ankle for about 10 seconds, and then do the same for the right ankle.

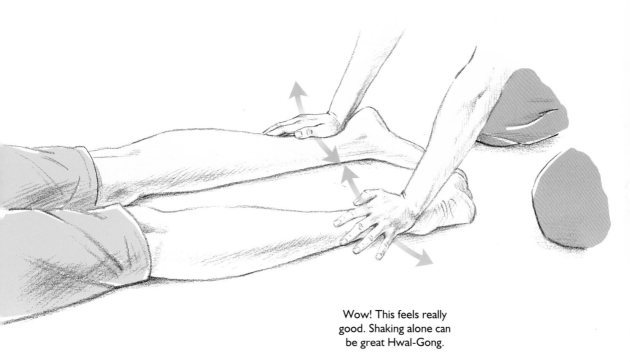

Wow! This feels really
good. Shaking alone can
be great Hwal-Gong.

3. Relaxing the Calf Muscles

Hwal-Gong Technique

Pressing with thumbs

Benefits

Good for relieving pain in the legs and lower back, and for relieving general fatigue. Also good for treating menstrual cramps, headaches, sciatica, and hernia.

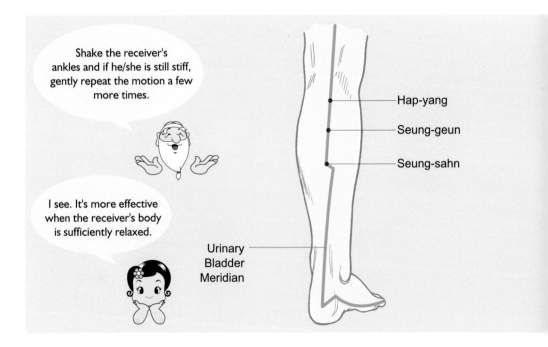

Shake the receiver's ankles and if he/she is still stiff, gently repeat the motion a few more times.

I see. It's more effective when the receiver's body is sufficiently relaxed.

Hap-yang

Seung-geun

Seung-sahn

Urinary Bladder Meridian

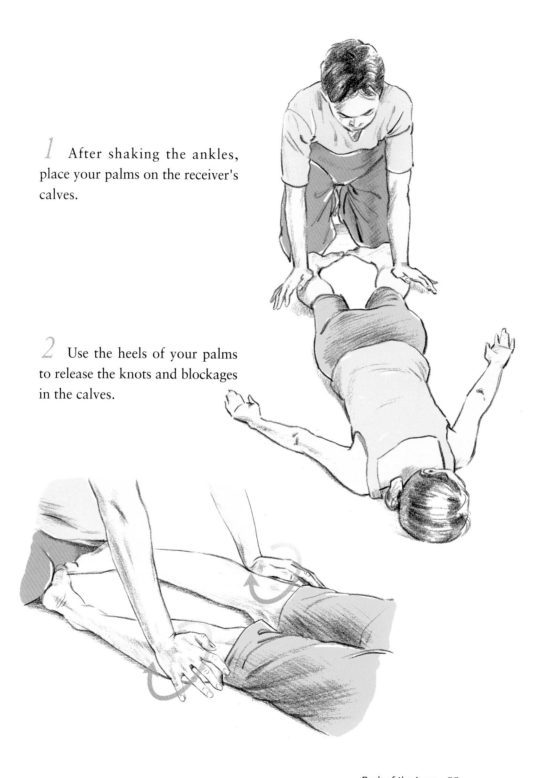

1 After shaking the ankles, place your palms on the receiver's calves.

2 Use the heels of your palms to release the knots and blockages in the calves.

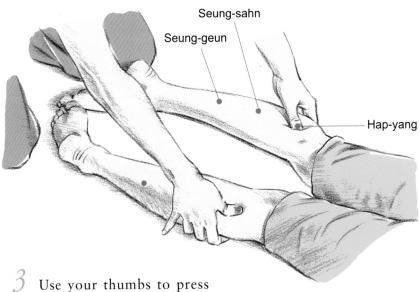

Seung-sahn

Seung-geun

Hap-yang

3 Use your thumbs to press along the midlines of the calves. Press the Hap-yang, Seung-geun, and Seung-sahn points.

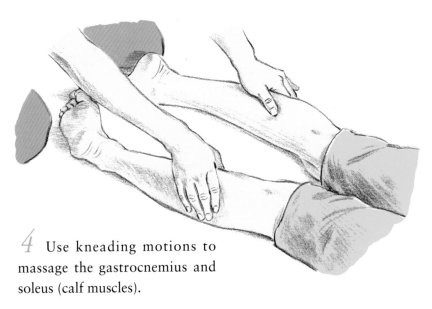

4 Use kneading motions to massage the gastrocnemius and soleus (calf muscles).

4. Relaxing the Posterior Sides of the Thighs

Hwal-Gong Technique

Pressing with palms

Benefits

Treats sciatica, fatigue, swollen hands and feet, pain in lower back and legs, and menopausal dysfunctions due to lack of exercise.

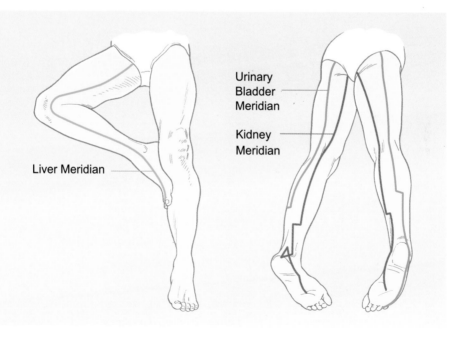

Liver Meridian

Urinary Bladder Meridian

Kidney Meridian

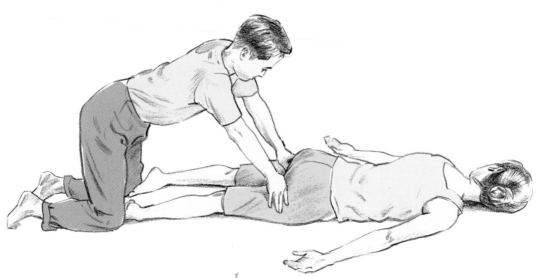

1 Kneel on the plantar surfaces of the receiver's feet and place your thumbs on the receiver's gluteal line (near ischial tuberosity).

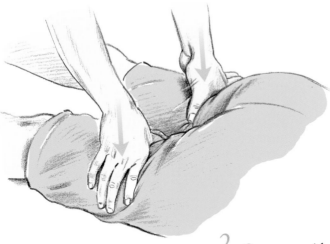

2 Compress with your palms gently below the gluteal muscles. Use body mechanics to shift weight on your upper body.

3 Press from below the gluteal muscles down to the heels of the feet and relax the legs.

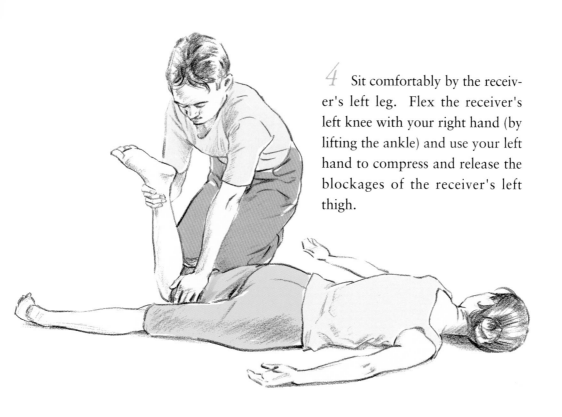

4 Sit comfortably by the receiver's left leg. Flex the receiver's left knee with your right hand (by lifting the ankle) and use your left hand to compress and release the blockages of the receiver's left thigh.

5 Knead the muscles on the lateral side of the thigh.

6 Do the same on the receiver's right leg.

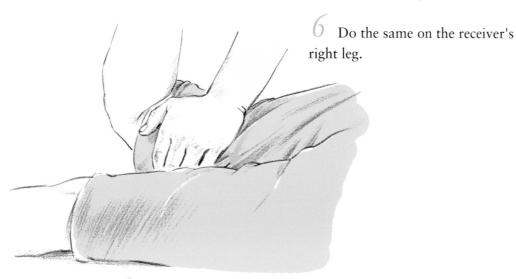

5. Elevating the Knees and Pressing the Thighs

Hwal-Gong Technique

Pressing with thumbs

Benefits

By promoting good circulation throughout the lower extremities, this technique helps to relieve fatigue quickly. This technique works especially well in conjunction with treatments for leg and waist pain.

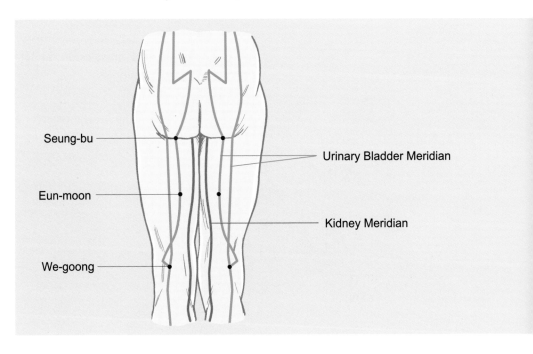

Seung-bu

Eun-moon

We-goong

Urinary Bladder Meridian

Kidney Meridian

When the giver
shifts positions, he/she
should do so gently
and subtly.

1 The giver should stand at the feet of the receiver, holding his/her ankles and allowing the knees to bend at a 90 ° angle.

2 Slowly shake the legs while keeping the legs bent, the shins vertical, and the knees almost touching the floor. Repeat ten times, and then gently lay down the legs on the floor.

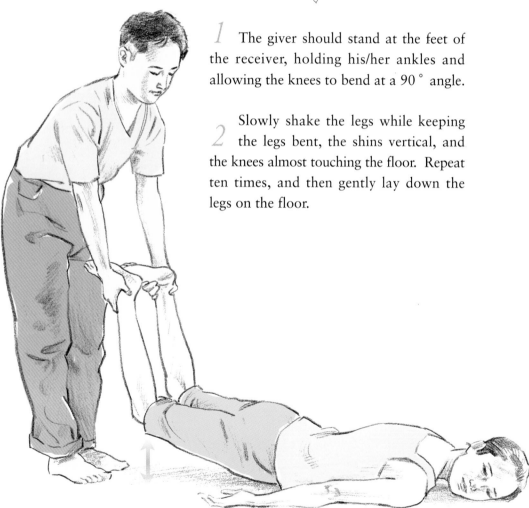

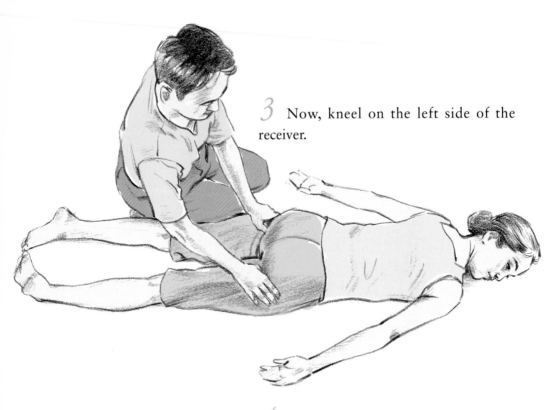

3 Now, kneel on the left side of the receiver.

4 Press along a straight line down the center of the thighs with your thumbs. Press the Seung-bu, Eun-moon, and We-joong points.

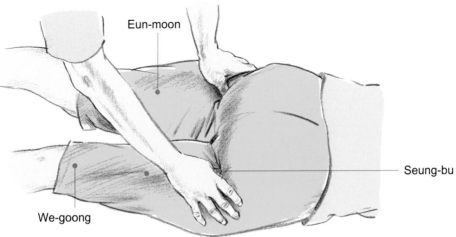

Eun-moon

Seung-bu

We-goong

96

6. Rubbing and Pressing the posterior of the Thighs

Hwal-Gong Techniques

Pressing with palms and shaking

Benefits

Stimulates the meridians related to the kidneys, urinary bladder and liver. Thus, it treats reproductive disordsers, lumbago, vertigo, tinnitus, fatigue, and vomiting.

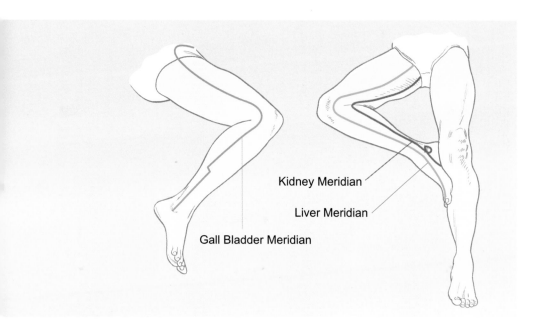

Kidney Meridian

Liver Meridian

Gall Bladder Meridian

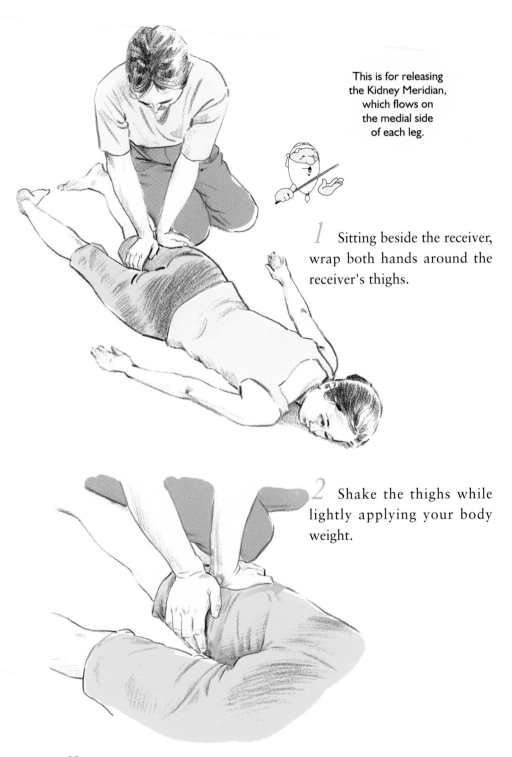

This is for releasing
the Kidney Meridian,
which flows on
the medial side
of each leg.

1 Sitting beside the receiver, wrap both hands around the receiver's thighs.

2 Shake the thighs while lightly applying your body weight.

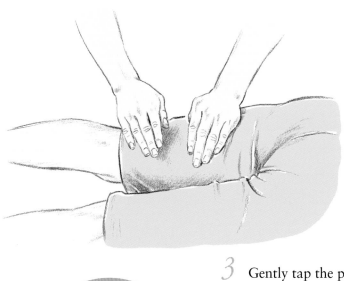

Use the following methods for tapping and finishing up.

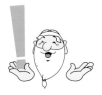

3 Gently tap the posterior surface of the receiver's thighs and smooth them out.

4 Cup your hands and gently tap the same area. The tapping may sound loud, but it should not cause pain.

5 Following the tapping, imagine that you are sweeping away stagnant energy by sweeping down from thighs to toes. Repeat tapping and sweeping.

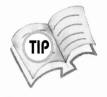

Rekindle the Flame:
Couple's Hwal-Gong

1. Blues Massage

Play comforting and romantic music and dance along.
Set the mood by incorporating appropriate scents and
lighting. Hold each other tightly, and melt away the
tension. Dancing like this for 10 to 20 minutes will
completely relieve your stress from a long day's work.

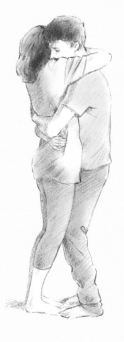

2. Sexual Dysfunction

Receiver should lie down and the giver should sit by
the receiver's side. The giver may use his/her palms to
press the receiver's pelvic area back and forth: the area
between Oh-chu–located 1 inch medial to the ASIS
(anterior superior iliac spine–the highest protrusion of
the hipbone lateral to the navel), and Gwan-won–located approximately 3 inches below the navel.

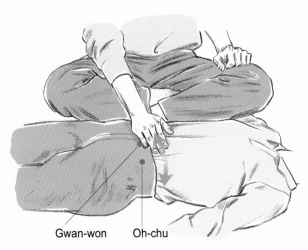

Gwan-won   Oh-chu

3. Tightening the Anus

1. Tightening your anus (muscles of the pelvic floor) stimulates the Im-maek (Conception Meridian) and Dok-maek (Governor Meridian), which, together, regulate the flow of your entire meridian system. Contracting the anus strengthens the reproductive sphincter muscles for women; it promotes good blood circulation, increases energy, and in general, builds resistance against stress.

1) Sit in a lotus or a half-lotus position. Alternatively, sit in a firm chair or stand up straight.

2) Push your lower abdomen forward and inhale, at the same time tightly contract your anus as much as you can.

3) Let your abdomen deflate while exhaling and relax the muscles.

4) Repeat this for three minutes. Doing this exercise three times a day–in the morning, noon, and evening–is especially effective.

4. Giving and Receiving Energy

1) You and your partner should lie down and form a continuous line.

2) Lift your legs with your knees bent at 90° angles. Let your feet touch your partner's soles.

3) Your palms should face up to receive energy and exchange your energy with your partner through the feet.

4) When you become used to this posture, raise both of your arms straight up with your palms facing up.

5) As you exhale through your mouth, expel negative energy through your Jang-shim (center of palm), while giving energy to your partner through Yong-chun (center of the sole).

* If it is difficult to lift your thighs, you may leave them down, and just let your soles touch your part-ner's soles.

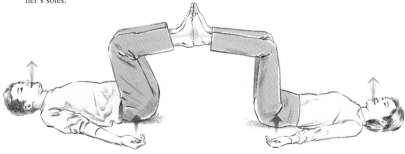

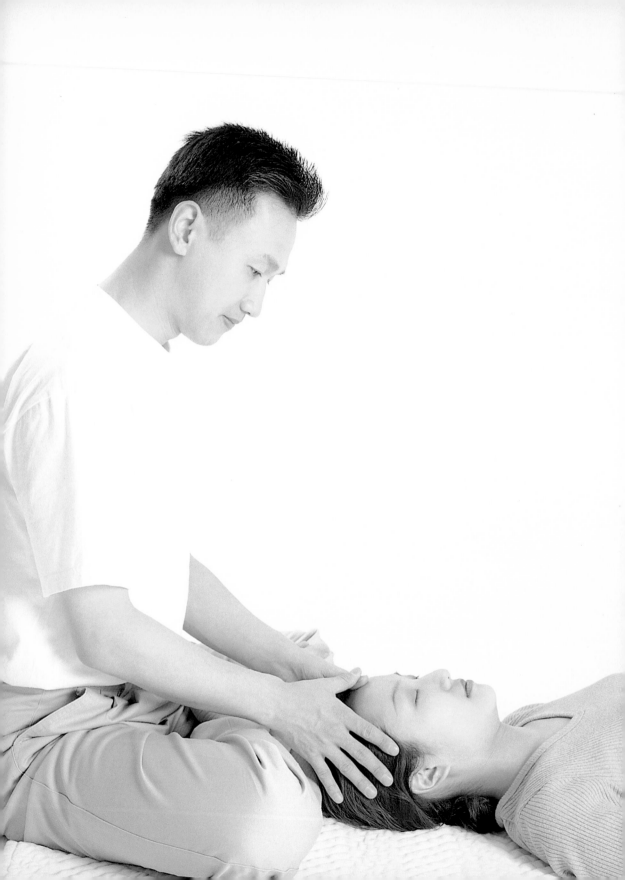

Chapter 6
Neck and Head

To receive Hwal-Gong
in a prone position
(stomach down), one would
need a thick mat and
a well-cushioned pillow.
Don't you think so?

If the legs are the pillars of our body, then the brain is the switch-board. The head is composed of tough cranial bones (the skull), and the brain. The brain is the most mysterious organ of the body. Nothing can be compared with the human brain.

Various meridian channels are branched out in the head. The head is the first place where Ki enters. Since it contains our switch-board, the brain, a good Hwal-Gong session on the head alone will bring relief to the entire body and wash away fatigue.

The neck is a passageway for respiration. The air we inhale pass-es through the neck and goes into our lungs, while its Ki-energy goes down to Dahn-jon. The neck is also susceptible to strain and burden due to bad habits and incorrect postures. Do not use your feet on the neck and shoulders: avoid applying excessive pressure when working on the neck and shoulders. These areas are very sensitive, and thus require special care. It is recommended that you use your thumbs or use gentle and light soothing strokes.

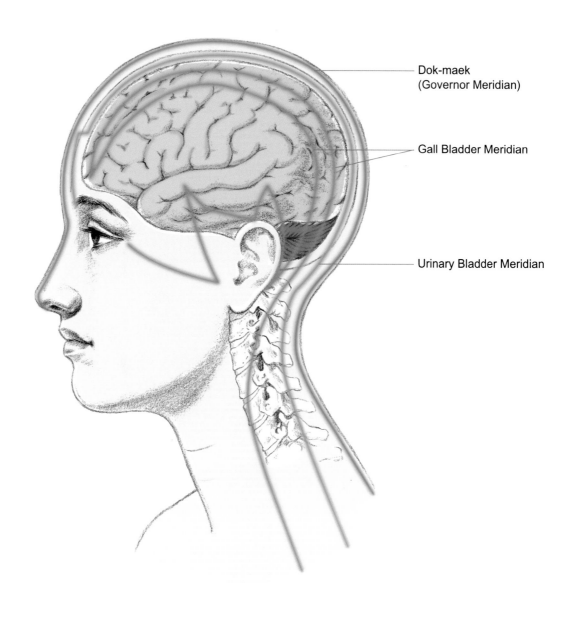

Dok-maek
(Governor Meridian)

Gall Bladder Meridian

Urinary Bladder Meridian

Meridians flowing on the neck and head

1. Pressing and Smoothing the Crown of the Head

Hwal-Gong Technique

Pressing with both thumbs overlapping, pressing with one thumb, smoothing with the palms.

Benefits

Good for headaches, eye problems, rhinitis, neuralgia, facial paralysis, insomnia, and ear problems.

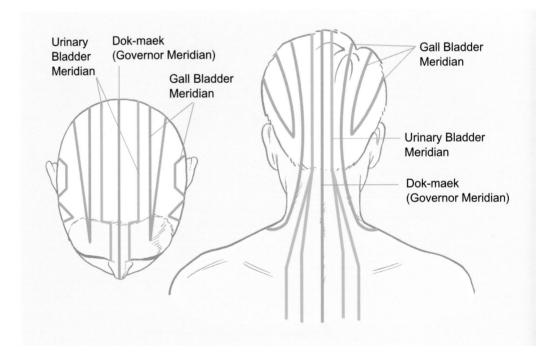

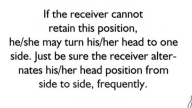

If the receiver cannot retain this position, he/she may turn his/her head to one side. Just be sure the receiver alternates his/her head position from side to side, frequently.

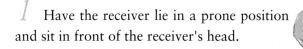

1   Have the receiver lie in a prone position and sit in front of the receiver's head.

2   From the crown of the head, overlap the thumbs and press along the Dok-maek (Governor Meridian).

3   Rotate the head to one side; support the head with one hand. Using the thumb of the other hand, press along the vertical line of the head about 1. 5 inches lateral to the middle of the head (along the Urinary Bladder Meridian).

4   Now, continue pressing with that thumb along the Gall Bladder Meridian (another 1. 5 inches lateral to the Urinary Bladder Meridian).

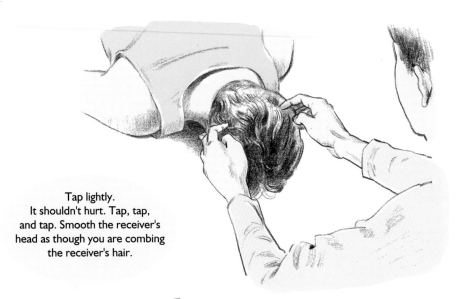

Tap lightly.
It shouldn't hurt. Tap, tap,
and tap. Smooth the receiver's
head as though you are combing
the receiver's hair.

5 Use the tips of your fingers (your fingerprinted side) to tap the entire head.

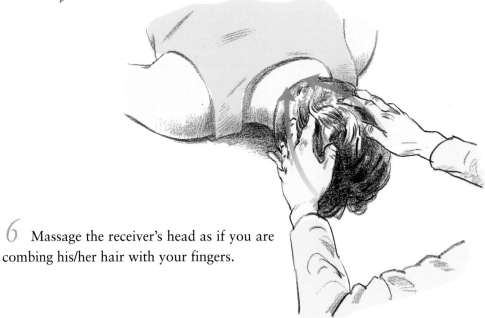

6 Massage the receiver's head as if you are
combing his/her hair with your fingers.

2. Relaxing and Pressing the Neck

Hwal-Gong Technique

Kneading with hands, pressing with thumbs

Benefits

Stimulating the Governor Meridian is beneficial for treating headaches, neck pains and vomiting. Stimulating the Urinary Bladder Meridian is good for headaches as well as for shoulder and back pains. Working on the Gall Bladder Meridian is good for muscleaches (from a cold), ear problems, and rhinitis.

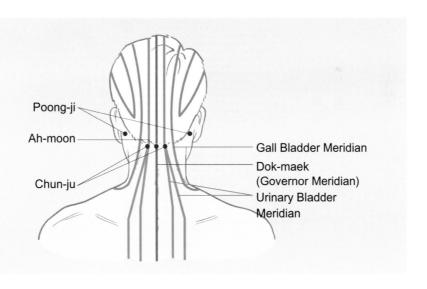

Poong-ji

Ah-moon

Chun-ju

Gall Bladder Meridian

Dok-maek
(Governor Meridian)

Urinary Bladder
Meridian

When rotating the receiver's head,
support it with both of your hands,
and move it carefully.

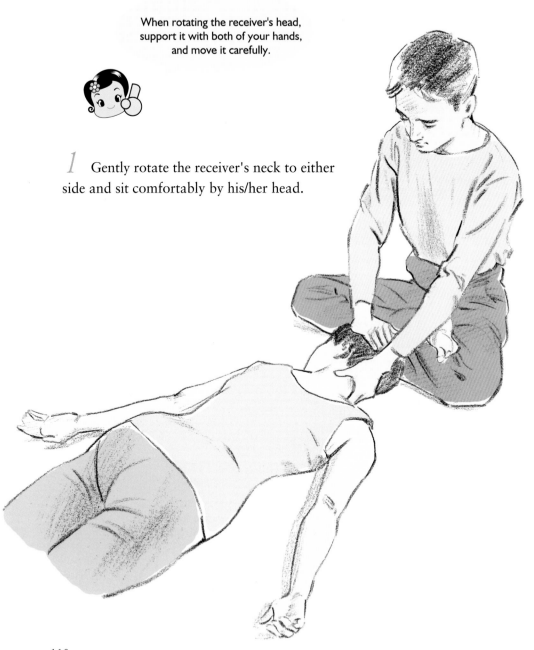

1 Gently rotate the receiver's neck to either side and sit comfortably by his/her head.

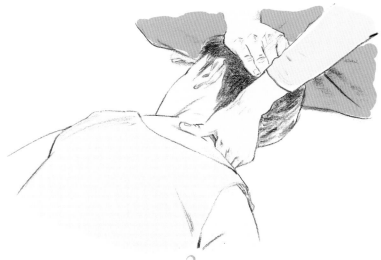

2 Lock the head in position by gently pressing it down with one hand. With your other hand, knead the nape of the neck.

3 Repeat this on the other side of the head.

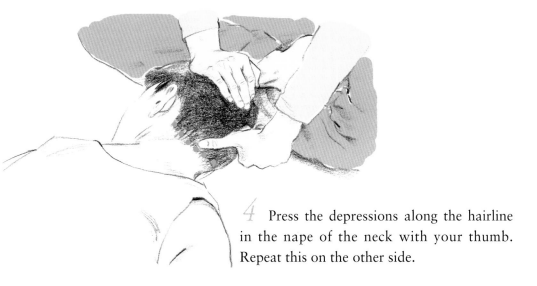

4 Press the depressions along the hairline in the nape of the neck with your thumb. Repeat this on the other side.

3. Stretching the Neck

Hwal-Gong Technique

Stretching with your hands

Benefits

Enhances blood supply to the Governor Meridian and enhances brain function. Relieves pain in neck, and helps to realign cervical vertebra. In general, this method is also effective for relieving fatigue and headaches.

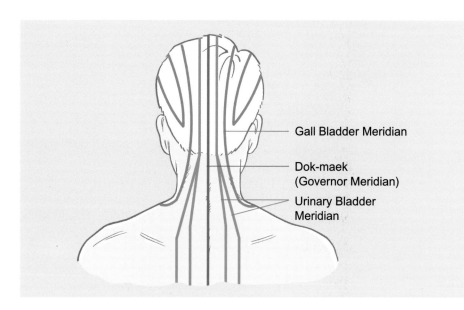

Gall Bladder Meridian

Dok-maek
(Governor Meridian)

Urinary Bladder
Meridian

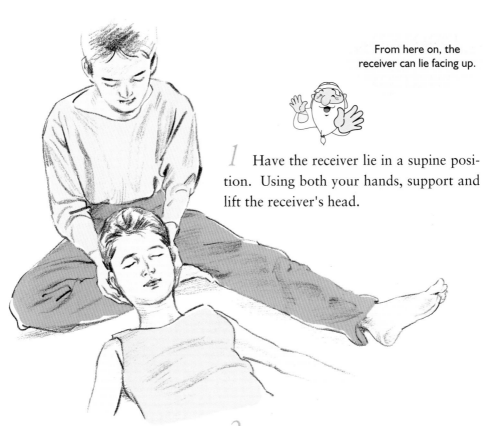

From here on, the receiver can lie facing up.

1 Have the receiver lie in a supine position. Using both your hands, support and lift the receiver's head.

2 Slowly and gently, rotate the receiver's head, alternating left and right.

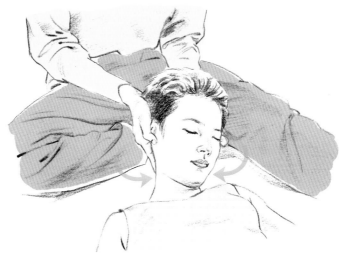

3 Cross your forearms
beneath the receiver's neck,
place your hands on his/her
shoulders and gently lift up
your arms.

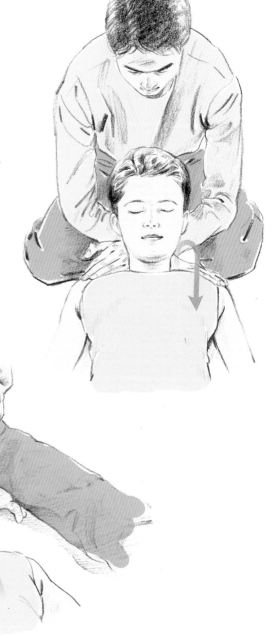

4 Gently wrap your hands
around the base of the receiver's head and pull it toward
you. It is recommended that
you pull it about 15° upwards.

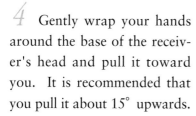

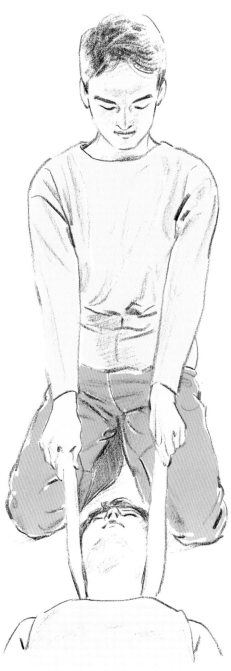

If your hands are slippery or tired, you may use a towel, instead.

5 Fold the towel lengthwise and place it under the receiver's neck. The receiver should hyperextend his/her neck. Begin stretching slightly, and gradually pull farther and farther (based on receiver's tolerance). Stretch for 1-3 minutes.

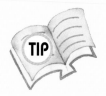

Getting Up on the Wrong Side of the Bed: Crick in the neck

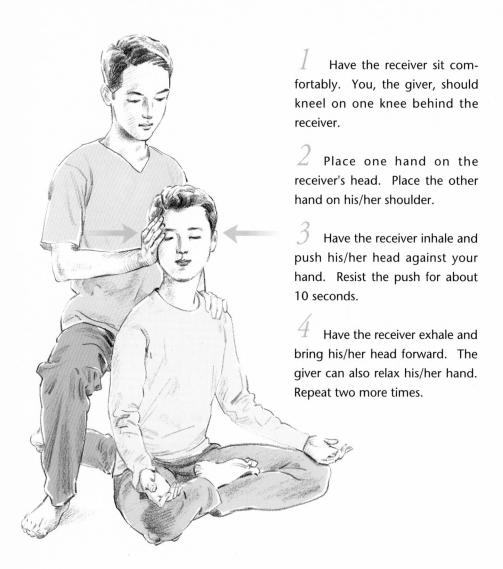

1   Have the receiver sit comfortably. You, the giver, should kneel on one knee behind the receiver.

2   Place one hand on the receiver's head. Place the other hand on his/her shoulder.

3   Have the receiver inhale and push his/her head against your hand. Resist the push for about 10 seconds.

4   Have the receiver exhale and bring his/her head forward. The giver can also relax his/her hand. Repeat two more times.

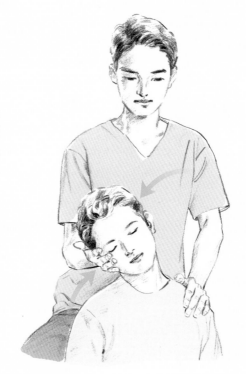

5   Now, have the receiver flex his/her neck toward the side and try to touch his/her shoulder on the same side. Push the receiver's head in the opposite direction.

6   As in the previous motion, have the receiver inhale on push and exhale on release. Repeat, alternating sides.

7   Repeat the previous method with the receiver's neck hyper-extended (bending backwards). Be cautious not to push too hard. Advise the receiver not to extend his/her neck too much or too abruptly. As before, inhale when you bend, and exhale on return.

4. Brain Hwal-Gong

Hwal-Gong Technique

Pulling and supporting with hands

Benefits

Calms nerves, relieves fatigue and stress, strengthens immune system, and helps relieve chronic headaches

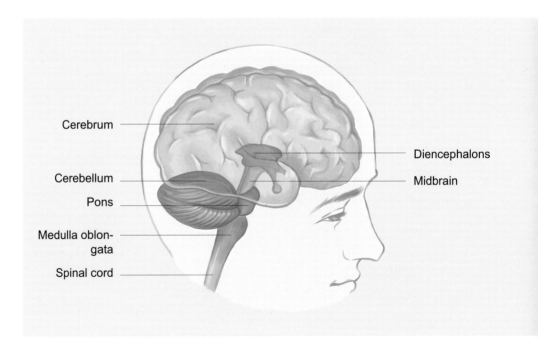

Cerebrum

Cerebellum

Pons

Medulla oblon-gata

Spinal cord

Diencephalons

Midbrain

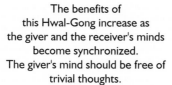

The benefits of
this Hwal-Gong increase as
the giver and the receiver's minds
become synchronized.
The giver's mind should be free of
trivial thoughts.

1 Before starting, the giver and the receiver are recommended to meditate to peaceful music.

2 Have the receiver lie in a supine position (lying on back), and sit by the receiver's head.

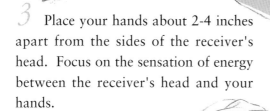

3 Place your hands about 2-4 inches apart from the sides of the receiver's head. Focus on the sensation of energy between the receiver's head and your hands.

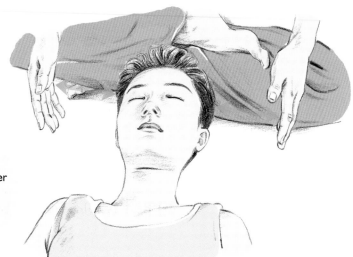

The head may feel
as though it is getting bigger
and smaller.
It might also feel soft,
mushy, or as if
it is vibrating.

4 If you feel like spreading out your hands, let your intuition guide as you spread them out. If you feel like bringing them together, bring them together.

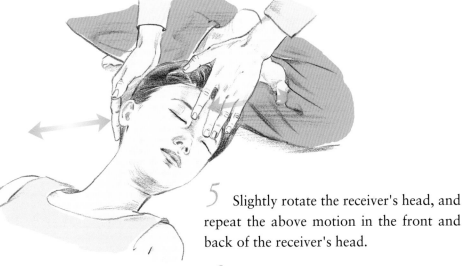

5 Slightly rotate the receiver's head, and repeat the above motion in the front and back of the receiver's head.

6 If the receiver falls asleep, allow him/her be to sleep for about 20 minutes.

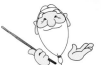

Wrap up the head and neck Hwal-Gong session like this.

1 When tension in the neck and shoulders is released, the receiver becomes relaxed enough to sleep. Support the receiver's head with Gyung-chim (Korean wooden pillow) or a rolled towel. Have the receiver's chin lifted slightly to allow his/her spine to be straight.

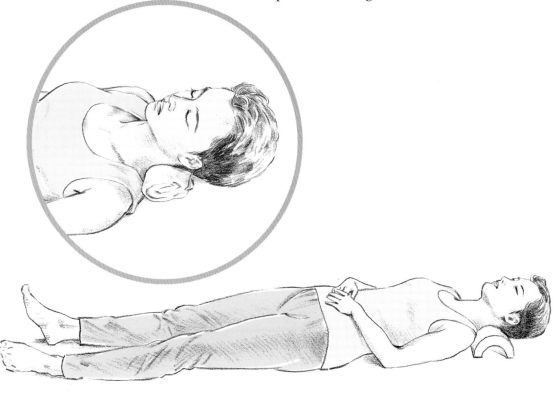

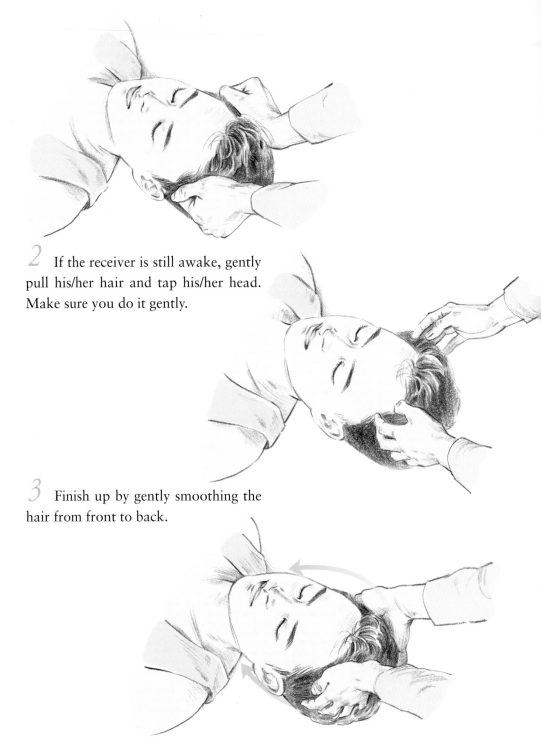

2   If the receiver is still awake, gently pull his/her hair and tap his/her head. Make sure you do it gently.

3   Finish up by gently smoothing the hair from front to back.

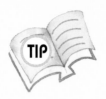

The Brain:
A Never Ending Puzzle

As you turn this page, do you wonder what goes on in your brain? The occipital lobe receives visual input and sends information to the frontal lobe. This information travels as a nerve cell to the tightly spread nervous tissue. Eventually, the information reaches the motor cortex.

The brain is responsible for receiving and interpreting information necessary for commanding and activating all bodily organs. The brain is responsible for producing sweat in the pores when hot and for constricting them when cold.

An average brain weighs about 3 lbs. , and uses . 75 liters of blood and 20-25% of our oxygen supply. A brain is as soft as tofu, and can easily be damaged. Therefore, it is protected by a hard skull. The front of the brain is called the cerebrum, which contains about 14 billion neurons. This area is where thought, judgment, creativity, and various functions, known as advanced mental activity, are processed. The wrinkly cerebrum is divided into the following lobes: frontal, parietal, temporal, and occipital lobes. Each of these lobes is responsible for reasoning, language, motor, auditory, and visual functions. The lower cerebrum controls our instinctive emotions and primitive urges.

Behind the cerebrum is the "small brain" called cerebellum. The cerebellum controls our balance. Between the cerebellum and the cerebrum is the thalamus, which can be considered a waiting area for all senses. Below the thalamus is the hypothalamus, which controls maintenances in our bodies. Below that, the midbrain regulates visual functions, while the medulla oblongata regulates vital functions. Together, the thalamus, midbrain, and medulla, are called the brain stem.

In this day and age, despite the technology we have to clone animals, the mysteries of the brain are still yet to be solved.

Improve Your Brain with Brain Gymnastics

1. Hold up one thumb at eye level in the center of your visual field, and draw an infinity sign.
2. Without moving your head, focus and follow your thumb with your eyes as you continue to draw this sign.
3. Repeat this exercise alternating thumbs.

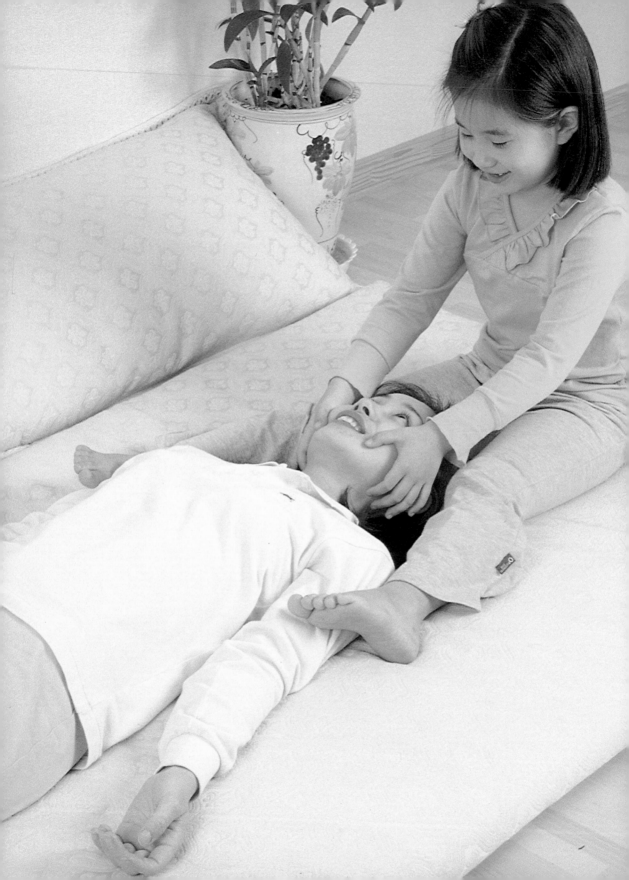

Chapter 7

Face

Unlike other animals, humans have a highly evolved frontal lobe. This gives us wide foreheads and wide parted eyebrows. Furthermore, each person has his/her unique appearance. A person's facial expression reflects not only their emotions but also his/her physical wellbeing. This is how the ancient art of facial diagnosis came about.

Each facial orifice is related to an organ, and reflects its condition. When you feel fatigued, your eyes become dim. This indicates the eye's relationship with the liver.

Similarly, many meridians are located on the face. These meridians include Large Intestine, Stomach, Small Intestine, Urinary Bladder, Triple Burner, Gall Bladder, Heart, Conception, and Governor Meridians. This means that facial Hwal-Gong can effectively address many symptoms.

Usually a person's first physical response to his/her physical or emotional discomfort is a frown. In just the opposite way, relaxing the face can elevate a person's mood and relax the entire body. Our faces can easily be relaxed, but it is important to work delicately and mind the details.

I'll pass on a priceless secret. One of the best and the most effective facial Hwal-Gong is laughing.

But wouldn't that create a lot of wrinkles around the eyes?

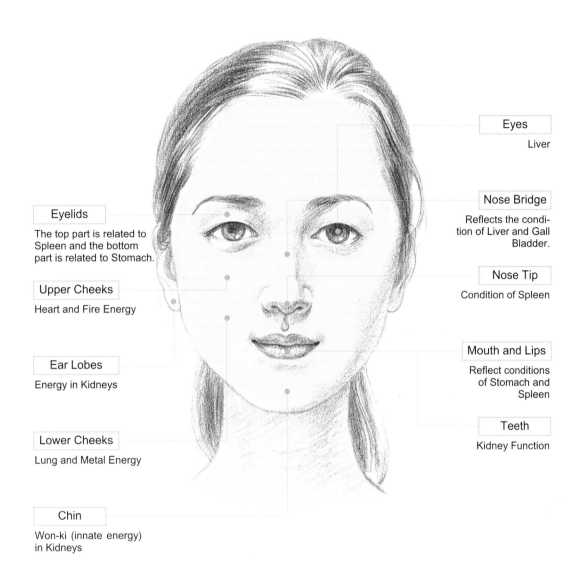

Eyes
Liver

Nose Bridge
Reflects the condition of Liver and Gall Bladder.

Nose Tip
Condition of Spleen

Eyelids
The top part is related to Spleen and the bottom part is related to Stomach.

Upper Cheeks
Heart and Fire Energy

Mouth and Lips
Reflect conditions of Stomach and Spleen

Teeth
Kidney Function

Ear Lobes
Energy in Kidneys

Lower Cheeks
Lung and Metal Energy

Chin
Won-ki (innate energy) in Kidneys

Relationship between facial features and internal organs

1. Facial Massage

Hwal-Gong Techniques

Pressing down with thumbs, tapping with fingers

Benefits

Treats headaches, facial pains, indigestion, toothaches, facial neuralgia, night blindness, frequent nose bleeds, and dermatological and esthetic benefits.

Do it as though you're smoothing over the entire facial meridian system.

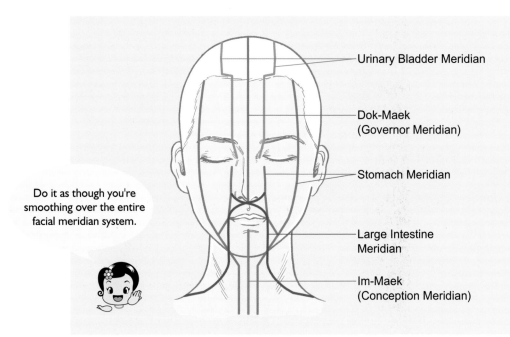

- Urinary Bladder Meridian
- Dok-Maek (Governor Meridian)
- Stomach Meridian
- Large Intestine Meridian
- Im-Maek (Conception Meridian)

First, apply Hwal-Gong over the facial muscles and meridians by gently massaging them with care.

The facial skin is sensitive, so it's a good idea to use massage oils, right?

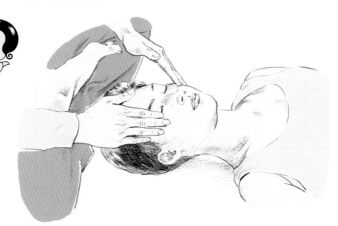

1 Have the receiver lie facing up, and sit by the receiver's head.

2 Massage the face by tugging the facial muscles upward. Pay attention to the meridians and muscles of the face. The facial skin is sensitive; therefore, you may need to use massage oil or other lubricants.

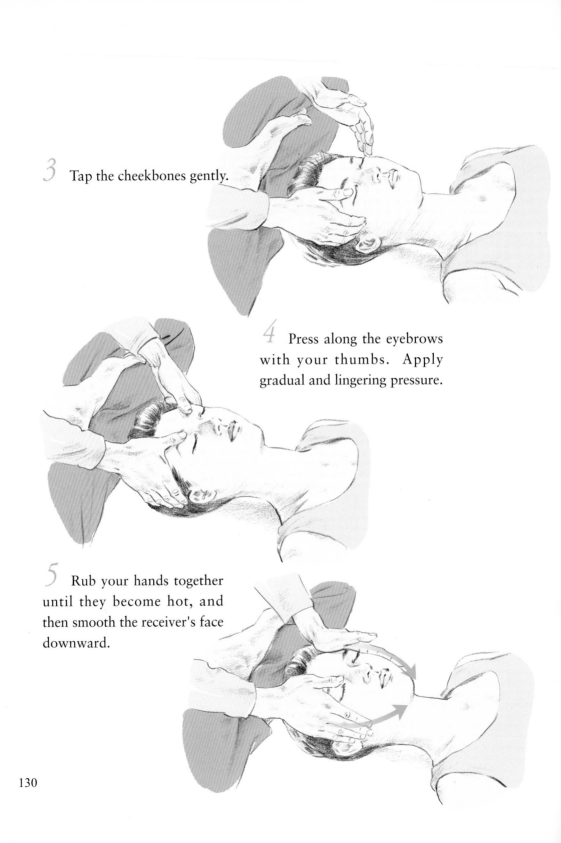

3   Tap the cheekbones gently.

4   Press along the eyebrows with your thumbs. Apply gradual and lingering pressure.

5   Rub your hands together until they become hot, and then smooth the receiver's face downward.

130

2. Facial Acupressure

Hwal-Gong Technique

Pressing with both thumbs

Benefits

Relieves fatigue, headaches, facial twitching, rhinitis, nasal congestion, fatigued eyes, tinnitus, ear problems, and tonsillitis.

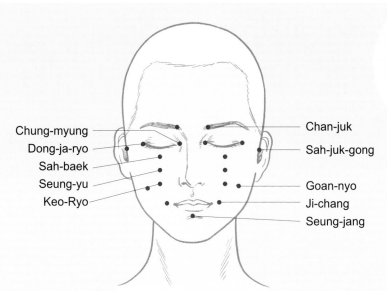

Acupressure on the face stimulates points in the Large Intestine, Stomach, Small Intestine, Urinary Bladder, and Triple Heater Meridians.

Chung-myung
Dong-ja-ryo
Sah-baek
Seung-yu
Keo-Ryo

Chan-juk
Sah-juk-gong
Goan-nyo
Ji-chang
Seung-jang

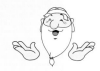

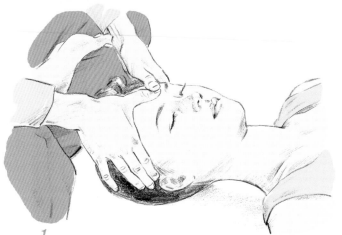

1 Overlap your thumbs, and glide them
laterally over the forehead.

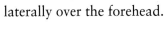

2 Starting from the temple press down
gently toward the center of the forehead
and back toward the temples.

3 Use your thumbs to apply gradual pressure on the temples, the depressions next to the eyebrows (Tae-yang point).

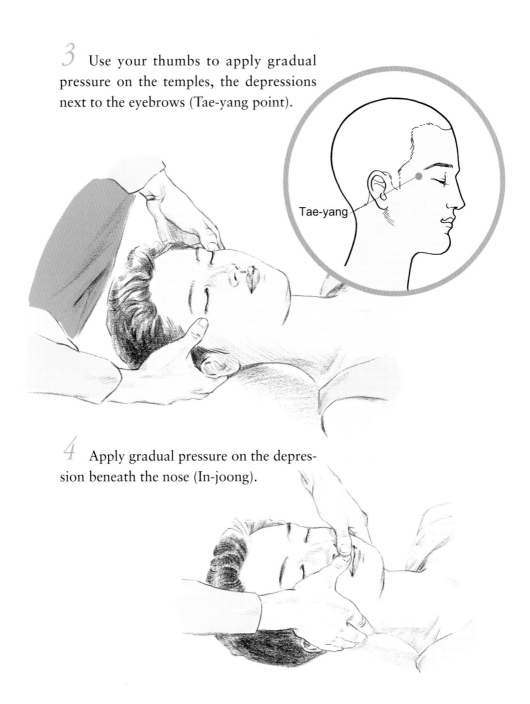

Tae-yang

4 Apply gradual pressure on the depression beneath the nose (In-joong).

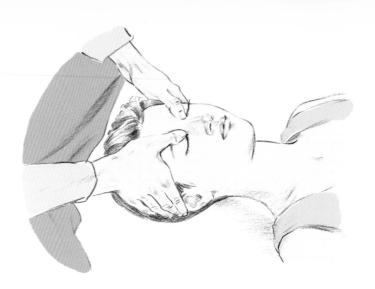

5 With your thumbs, press around the
entire orbit starting from the upper medial
corners of the eyes.

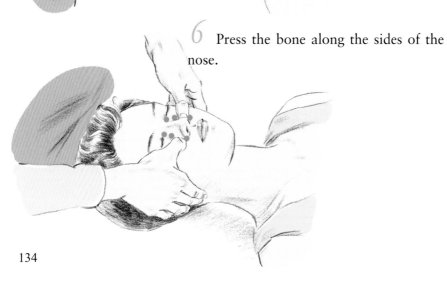

6 Press the bone along the sides of the
nose.

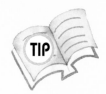

Self-Massage:
Relieving Fatigue in the Eyes I

It is recommended that you do this exercise after reading or whenever your eyes feel strained. This exercise is effective because the palms emanate natural healing energy. However, it is not necessary to press the palms directly on the eyes or eyelids.

Palms-on-Eyes Exercise
1. Rub your hands together until hot, and then place them lightly over your eyes.
2. With your eyes covered, look up, down, left and right. Turn them clockwise and counter-clock wise, three times each. Imagine that your eyes are following a moving object.

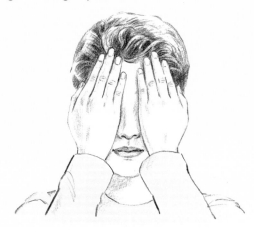

Water Immersion Eye Exercise
1. Fill a washbasin or sink, and immerse your face in the water. In that position, move your eyes up, down, left and right three times.
2. Turn your eyes clockwise and counter-clock wise three times each.
3. Try hot-and-cold therapy. Prepare two basins, one with warm to hot water and the other with cold. Immerse your face for five minutes in one basin, and then the other. This is recommended in the morning and night or after an outing.

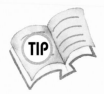

Self-Massage:
Relieving Fatigue in the Eyes II

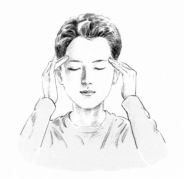

Pressing around the Eyes

1 Close your eyes, and gently press around your eyes with your fingertips. Increase the pressure to your desire, and hold the pressure for 2-3 seconds.

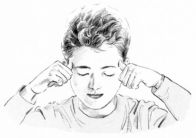

2 Press your temples with your thumbs. Continue pressing, and each time hold the pressure for about one second.

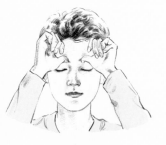

3 Use your thumbs to press down on your Chan-juk points (medial corners of the eyebrows). Hold the pressure each time as you continue pressing in circular motions. Finish by pressing slightly upward. Do the same for Chung-myung points (medial corners of eyes).

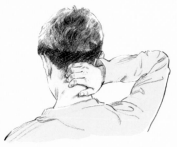

4 Since the occipital lobe of the brain, which regulates vision, is around the nape of the neck, it is good to massage this area.

3. Releasing the Jaw Joints (TMJ)

Hwal-Gong Technique

Pressing with fingers and thumbs

Benefits

Treats toothaches, jaw pain (TMJ inflammation), ear problems

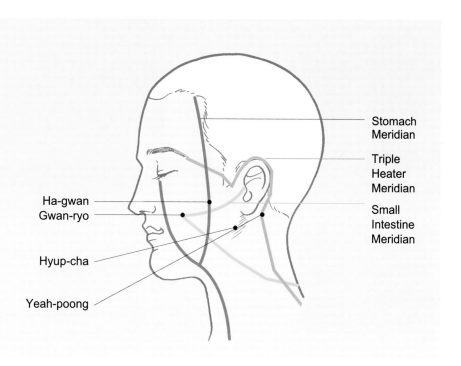

Ha-gwan
Gwan-ryo

Hyup-cha

Yeah-poong

Stomach Meridian

Triple Heater Meridian

Small Intestine Meridian

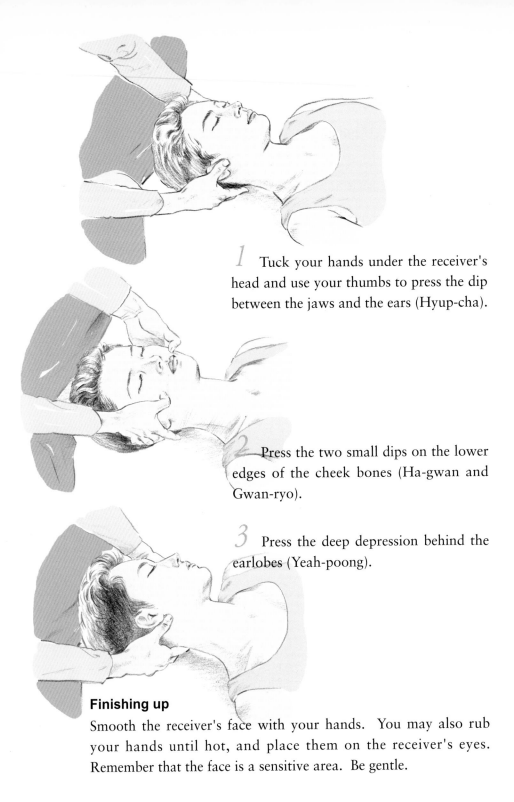

1   Tuck your hands under the receiver's head and use your thumbs to press the dip between the jaws and the ears (Hyup-cha).

2   Press the two small dips on the lower edges of the cheek bones (Ha-gwan and Gwan-ryo).

3   Press the deep depression behind the earlobes (Yeah-poong).

Finishing up

Smooth the receiver's face with your hands. You may also rub your hands until hot, and place them on the receiver's eyes. Remember that the face is a sensitive area. Be gentle.

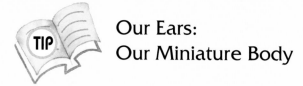

Our Ears:
Our Miniature Body

Just pulling one's hair gently is an effective Hwal-Gong technique, pulling one's ears is tremendously beneficial. Look carefully at an ear, and you will see the shape of a fetus (with its head by the earlobe and legs by the top of the ear). Treating various illnesses as well as anesthetizing by applying acupuncture on the ears has long been practiced by Eastern medicine.

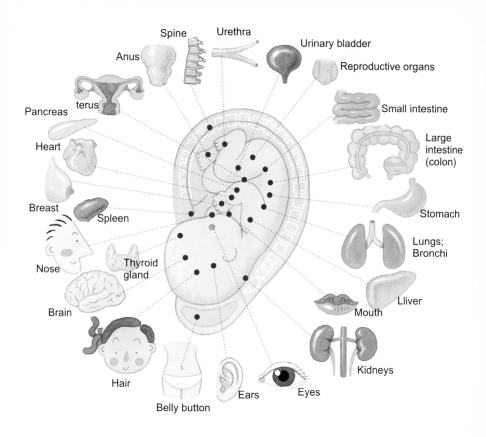

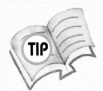

Symptom-specific Tips for Ear Hwal-Gong

Diet

Press the center of the bridge of an ear (above the auditory meatus) with your middle finger. Slowly pull the top part of the ear and earlobe.

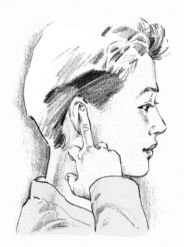

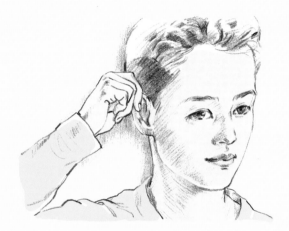

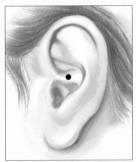

For diet

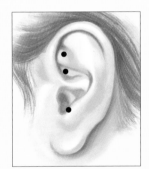

To relieve constipation

Stress

Fold an ear with the edge of your hand (the little finger side), and gently rub it.

Dim Eyes

Grab an earlobe with your thumb and an index finger, and press while gently pulling it.

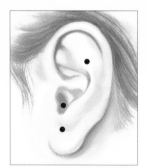

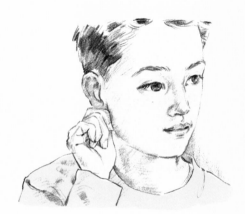

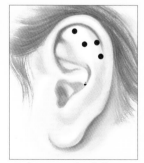

to quit smoking

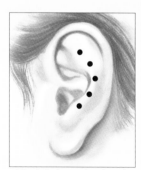

Improve circulation

Alleviate lower back pain

Hwal-Gong Classified by Symptoms

Abdominal cramps_72

Back pain_109, 112

Bronchitis_59

Colon dysfunctions_59

Constipation_59, 69, 140

Diabetes_72

Diarrhea_69, 72

Diet_140

Ear problems_106, 109, 131, 137

Eczema_67

Eye problems_106

Facial neuralgia_128

Facial pains_128

Facial paralysis_106

Facial twitching_131

Fatigue_63, 67, 69, 82, 88, 91, 94, 112, 118, 131

Fatigued eyes_131

Frozen shoulders_57, 59

Headache_88, 106, 109, 112, 118, 128, 131

Hernia_88

Hypertension_57

Improve circulation_141

Indigestion_59, 128

Insomnia_106

Irregular menstruation_69

Jaw pain_(TMJ inflammation) 137

Leukorrhea_67

Lower back pain_67, 88, 91, 141

Lumbago_97

Menopausal dysfunction_91

Menstrual cramps_67, 86

Muscleaches_109

Nasal congestion_131

Neck pain_88, 109

Neck tension_57

Neuralgia_106

Night blindness_128

Nose bleeds_128

Pain in legs_91

Pneumonia_59

Reproductive disorder_97

Rhinitis_106, 109, 131

Sciatica_67, 69, 72, 88, 91

Shoulder pain_59, 109

Stiff neck_86

Stomach dysfunctions_59, 63

Stomachache_72

Stress_118

Swollen hands and feet_91

Tinnitus_97, 131

To quit smoking_141

Tonsillitis_131

Toothaches_128

Vomiting_97, 109

142